EDUCAT
ROYAL IN
D0476856

Human Disease for Dentists

BLACKBURN EDUCATION CENTRE
LIBRARY

TB07333

Human Disease for Dentists

Edited by

Professor David J. Gawkrodger
MD, FRCP, FRCPE
Consultant Dermatologist and
Honorary Professor of Dermatology,
University of Sheffield,
Royal Hallamshire Hospital,
Sheffield, UK

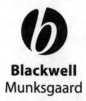

Blackwell
Munksgaard

⌐CATION CENTRℇ
LIBRARY
ACC. No: TBO7333
CLASS No: 617. 6 HUM

© 2004 by Blackwell Munksgaard, a Blackwell Publishing company

Editorial offices:
Blackwell Publishing Ltd, 9600 Garsington Road, Oxford OX4 2DQ, UK
  Tel: +44 (0) 1865 776868
Blackwell Publishing Professional, 2121 State Avenue, Ames, Iowa 50014-8300, USA
  Tel: +1 515 292 0140
Blackwell Munksgaard, 1, Rosenørns Allé, P.O. Box 227, DK-1502 Copenhagen V, Denmark
  Tel: +45 77 33 33 33
Blackwell Science Asia Pty Ltd, 550 Swanston Street, Carlton, Victoria 3053, Australia
  Tel: +61 (0)3 8359 1011

The right of the Authors to be identified as the Authors of this Work has been asserted in accordance with the Copyright, Designs and Patents Act 1988.

All rights reserved. No part of this publication may be reproduced, stored in a retrieval system, or transmitted, in any form or by any means, electronic, mechanical, photocopying, recording or otherwise, except as permitted by the UK Copyright, Designs and Patents Act 1988, without the prior permission of the publisher.

First published 2004 by Blackwell Munksgaard, a Blackwell Publishing Company

Library of Congress Cataloging-in-Publication Data
Human disease for dentists / edited by David J. Gawkrodger.
    p. ; cm.
Includes bibliographical references and index.
    ISBN 0-632-06453-6 (pbk. : alk. paper)
    1. Diagnosis. 2. Diseases. 3. Dentists.
    [DNLM: 1. Clinical Medicine – methods. 2. Dental Care – methods.
WB 102 H918 2004] I. Gawkrodger, D.J. (David J.)

RC71.3.H85 2004
616–dc22   2003022526

ISBN 0-632-06453-6

A catalogue record for this title is available from the British Library

Set in 11/13pt Trump Mediaeval
by Graphicraft Limited, Hong Kong
Printed and bound in India
by Replika Press Pvt. Ltd, Kundli 131028

The publisher's policy is to use permanent paper from mills that operate a sustainable forestry policy, and which has been manufactured from pulp processed using acid-free and elementary chlorine-free practices. Furthermore, the publisher ensures that the text paper and cover board used have met acceptable environmental accreditation standards.

For further information on Blackwell Munksgaard, visit our website:
www.dentistry.blackwellmunksgaard.com

EDUCATION CENTRE LIBRARY
ROYAL INFIRMARY, BLACKBURN

Contents

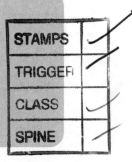

STAMPS

TRIGGER

CLASS

SPINE

Contributors

David J. Gawkrodger MD FRCP FRCPE
Consultant Dermatologist, Royal Hallamshire Hospital, Sheffield S10 2JF and Honorary Professor of Dermatology, University of Sheffield.

Narjot S. Ahluwalia BM MRCPsych
Clinical Lecturer in Psychiatry, University of Sheffield, Northern General Hospital, Sheffield S5 7AU.

Mohammed Akil MD FRCP
Consultant Rheumatologist, Royal Hallamshire Hospital, Sheffield S10 2JF.

Paul B. Anderson BM FRCP
Consultant Physician, Northern General Hospital, Sheffield S5 7AU.

Maria Asensio MB MMedSci
Specialist Registrar in Medical Microbiology, Northern General Hospital, Sheffield S5 7AU.

Sylvia M. Bates MB MRCOG
Specialist Registrar in Genito-Urinary Medicine, Royal Hallamshire Hospital, Sheffield S10 2JF.

Steve R. Brennan MB FRCP
Consultant Physician, Northern General Hospital, Sheffield S5 7AU.

Lynne Caddick MB MRCP
Consultant Physician, Royal Hallamshire Hospital, Sheffield S10 2JF.

Kevin Channer MD FRCP
Consultant Cardiologist, Royal Hallamshire Hospital, Sheffield S10 2JF.

Abdel Meguid El Nahas PhD FRCP
Professor of Renal Medicine, University of Sheffield, Northern General Hospital, Sheffield S5 7AU.

Fiona M. Fairlie MD MRCOG
Consultant Obstetrician, Jessop Wing, Royal Hallamshire Hospital, Sheffield S10 2JF.

Sheila M. Fairlie BDS
General Dental Practitioner, c/o Jessop Wing, Royal Hallamshire Hospital, Sheffield S10 2JF.

Iftikhar U. Haq MD MRCP
Consultant Cardiologist, Royal Victoria Infirmary, Newcastle-Upon-Tyne NE1 4LP.

Jane Holmes DipCOT
Senior Occupational Therapist, Royal Hallamshire Hospital, Sheffield S10 2JF.

Peter R. Jackson PhD FRCP
Reader in Clinical Pharmacology, University of Sheffield, Royal Hallamshire Hospital, Sheffield S10 2JF.

Darren A. Kilroy MB FRCSE
Specialist Registrar in Accident and Emergency Medicine, Northern General Hospital, Sheffield S5 7AU.

Graham Knight MB FRCP
Consultant Physician, Rotherham District General Hospital, Rotherham S60 2UD.

Rod Lawson PhD MRCP
Consultant Respiratory Physician, Royal Hallamshire Hospital, Sheffield S10 2JF.

Mark McAlindon DM FRCP
Consultant Gastroenterologist, Royal Hallamshire Hospital, Sheffield S10 2JF.

Andrew J.G. McDonagh MB FRCP
Consultant Dermatologist, Royal Hallamshire Hospital, Sheffield S10 2JF.

Mike Makris MD MRCPath
Senior Clinical Lecturer in Haematology, University of Sheffield, Royal Hallamshire Hospital, Sheffield S10 2JF.

Gary H. Mills MB FRCA
Senior Clinical Lecturer in Anaesthetics, University of Sheffield,
Royal Hallamshire Hospital, Sheffield S10 2JF.

Patrick Mitchell MB FRCS
Specialist Registrar in Neurosurgery, Royal Hallamshire Hospital,
Sheffield S10 2JF.

John D.C. Newell-Price MB MRCP
Senior Clinical Lecturer in Endocrinology, University of Sheffield,
Northern General Hospital, Sheffield S5 7AU.

Somdutt Prasad MS FRCSE
Consultant Ophthalmologist, Arrowe Park Hospital, The Wirral,
CH49 5PE.

John E. Peacock MB FRCA
Consultant in Pain Management, Royal Hallamshire Hospital,
Sheffield S10 2JF.

Robert C. Read MD FRCP
Professor of Infectious Diseases, University of Sheffield, Royal
Hallamshire Hospital, Sheffield S10 2JF.

Johnny J. Ross MB FRCA
Senior Clinical Lecturer in Anaesthetics, University of Sheffield,
Northern General Hospital, Sheffield S5 7AU.

Phil S. Sanmuganathan MB MRCP
Lecturer in Stroke Medicine, Western Infirmary, Glasgow G11
6NT.

Basil Sharrack PhD FRCP
Consultant Neurologist, Royal Hallamshire Hospital, Sheffield S10
2JF.

Helen Till RGN
Instructor in Resuscitation, Royal Hallamshire Hospital, Sheffield
S10 2JF.

David Turnbull BM FRCA
Specialist Registrar in Anaesthetics, Royal Hallamshire Hospital,
Sheffield S10 2JF.

John Winfield MB FRCP
Consultant Physician in Rheumatology, Royal Hallamshire
Hospital, Sheffield S10 2JF.

Mark P.J. Yardley MPhil FRCSE
Consultant ENT Surgeon, Royal Hallamshire Hospital, Sheffield
S10 2JF.

Wilf W. Yeo MD FRCP
Senior Clinical Lecturer in Clinical Pharmacology, University of
Sheffield, Royal Hallamshire Hospital, Sheffield S10 2JF.

Preface

Dental surgeons require skills in medicine to treat their patients effectively. They need to be able to assess any medical condition when the patient is lying in the dental chair, so that any one who may be at particular risk or who needs special consideration is recognised and treated appropriately. Examples include patients with heart problems, women who are pregnant or subjects with a history of psychiatric disorder. Some dental problems are a part of the patient's general medical condition and the dentist should recognise this, e.g. the dry mouth in Sjogren's syndrome related to rheumatoid arthritis, or abnormalities of the dentition in acromegaly.

Dentists are called upon to deal with medical emergencies from time to time. This means they need to be familiar with, for example, cardiopulmonary resuscitation, the management of diabetic problems or an attack of asthma, and coping with fits and collapses.

Many patients, especially the elderly, are on drugs for a variety of conditions and it is vital that the dental surgeon knows something of the pharmacology of these medications and how they might interact with drugs that the dentist may use. Anticoagulants, immunosuppressive agents and antihypertensive medication are important examples. The use of local anaesthetics is central to dentistry and dentists should have an in-depth knowledge of anaesthetics in general, including perioperative care.

The generic skills of taking and recording a history are familiar to dental students by the time they reach the part of their course in which they learn about human disease, but the skills concerned with obtaining a medical history and making a basic clinical general medical examination, even of a clothed patient, will need to be learnt. The ability to elicit, recognise and interpret basic physical signs of human disease is of considerable benefit to the dentist and his or her patient when a medical problem supervenes.

In this book the editor and contributors aim to provide a guide to human disease for dental students, qualified dentists, and health workers associated with dentistry. The work is focused on the requirements of the dental profession and is not a mini medical textbook. Conditions that the dentist is unlikely to come across are not included. The book is structured to start with the skills of history taking and basic examination, and moves on to a clinical section covering the major systemic diseases and a section on pharmacology and anaesthetics as applied to dentistry.

Finally, specifically but not exclusively for those taking examinations, a 'revision' section comprises a problem-based learning format to illustrate some of the problems that may occur in dental practice, a selection of colour photographs with captions, illustrating conditions covered in the text, some multiple choice questions, and a short-answer question exam paper.

I hope the reader will like the book and that the objective of achieving a sound skill and knowledge base in human disease, along side the necessary clinical experience, will be realised. Every book has its strengths and weaknesses and I should be grateful to receive comments on how this volume might be improved.

David J. Gawkrodger
Sheffield

Acknowledgements

The preparation of this book came out of a commitment to organising the 'Human diseases' course at the Dental School of the University of Sheffield. The editor is grateful to the lecturers, whose timely contributions were central to the project, and thanks Professor Tim Higenbottam, senior coordinator for the course, Professor Colin Smith and Professor Alan Brook, deans of the School of Dentistry, University of Sheffield, and Professor Frank Woods, Head of the Section of Clinical Science, for support and encouragement.

Mr. Keith Smith and Dr. Tilly Loescher, senior clinical lecturers in Oral and Maxillofacial Surgery, University of Sheffield, kindly reviewed the manuscript and provided many helpful comments.

The secretarial assistance of Mrs. Gillian Sykes and Mrs. Pat Bruce are gratefully acknowledged. The support of Ms. Caroline Connelly, Ms. Emma Lonie and Mr. Richard Miles on behalf of the publishers, Blackwell Munksgaard, is appreciated.

CHAPTER 1
Taking a Medical History

Dental practitioners should be able to take an adequate medical history from their patients to pre-empt problems that may arise during dental treatment. Taking a history in dental and medical practice also includes developing a rapport with patients, to engender mutual trust, which is the cornerstone of the practitioner–patient relationship.

This chapter outlines a standard approach to history taking in medicine and surgery that focuses on the specific requirements of a dentist. The aims of taking such a history are:

• to obtain an accurate sequential account of the presenting symptoms to create a differential diagnosis
• to ask specific questions to focus and corroborate the most likely diagnosis
• to assess whether complications have occurred on the basis of associated symptoms
• to put the medical problem into context, by knowledge of the patient's past medical and social history.

Some dental students believe that only the past medical history – and perhaps drug treatment – are important in dental practice. However, the General Dental Council and examiners in medical and surgical subjects expect dental students to be proficient in history taking, clinical skills and knowledge, so that when they are qualified dental practitioners they can deal with medical emergencies that may occur in the dental chair.

Patient's details

At the start of every history you should introduce yourself and explain the purpose of the consultation. Bedside manner is a very personal characteristic, but courtesy, patience, allowing patients to tell their own story, and being aware of their fears and expectations are qualities you should aim for.

You will need to record the patient's name, age, sex and occupation, as well as the date, time and place of consultation. It is common practice to document who referred the patient, and whether they were seen as an emergency. Once these details are complete, the consultation can begin by eliciting the presenting complaint. This is the main problem that has made the patient seek medical attention.

The presenting complaint (PC)

The presenting complaint (or complaints) is the most important part of the history. It should be documented clearly as a single phrase or sentence that summarises the main symptom. For example a presenting complaint might be 'chest pain' or 'shortness of breath' or 'loss of consciousness'. If there is more than one complaint these should be listed separately as each may require a history of the presenting complaint.

Resist the temptation to write the entire history in this section as it can be difficult to pick out specific complaints from a long paragraph of prose. You should also resist writing down someone else's diagnosis as the presenting complaint. For example 'the patient presents with a myocardial infarction' (MI). The diagnosis may be incorrect and it is best to approach every new patient with a completely open mind.

In dental practice there are certain presenting complaints that should sound alarm bells as they may signal the possibility of a medical emergency occurring in the dental chair. These would include:

- chest pain
- palpitations
- shortness of breath
- loss of consciousness
- wheezing
- bruising or bleeding tendency
- jaundice
- joint pains
- some skin rashes

Other presenting complaints may be important because they lie between the boundaries of dental and medical practice, for example:

- headache, earache or facial pain
- new lesions in the mouth or face
- swellings in the neck

The history of presenting complaint (HPC)

For each presenting complaint or problem you need to establish the course of events. You may wish to ask the patient when they were last well, and then record the development of symptoms chronologically. Essential features of the history of each presenting complaint would be:

- the onset (and perhaps offset) of symptoms
- the duration of the complaint
- any relieving or exacerbating (worsening) factors including treatments
- any associated symptoms
- the pattern of the complaint, e.g. whether continuous or recurrent episodes.

At the end of the history of the presenting complaint it should be possible to form an idea of the differential diagnosis (the most likely possibilities), and perhaps to have accrued sufficient evidence from the history to focus very strongly on one particular diagnosis. Despite the availability of an extensive array of fancy investigations, 80% of the evidence supporting a diagnosis is still obtained from the history.

Here are three examples of typical histories that may be obtained from the same presenting complaint, 'loss of consciousness', giving totally different diagnoses.

Example 1

Sudden episode of loss of consciousness this morning while shopping
- known insulin-dependent diabetic
- did not have breakfast this morning as woke up late
- had usual dose of insulin 34 units of Humulin I
- episode lasted 30 minutes until brought to Accident and Emergency
- complete recovery after dextrose infusion
- two previous episodes in last four weeks since dose of insulin increased
- no other symptoms or complaints

Most likely diagnosis: hypoglycaemic episode

Example 2

Sudden episode of loss of consciousness this morning while shopping
- remembers feeling odd before it happened, as if not his usual self
- cannot remember anything else until waking up in hospital

- feels very drowsy
- noticed that he had been incontinent of urine when he woke up in hospital
- sore left side of tongue and bleeding mouth (suggests tongue biting)
- friend reports rhythmical shaking of limbs while unconscious
- no previous episodes

Most likely diagnosis: epileptic grand mal convulsion (possible first attack)

Example 3

Sudden episode of loss of consciousness this morning while shopping
- started with an attack of chest pain like her usual angina
- pain central and crushing, radiating down left arm and up to jaw
- pain lasted 15 minutes
- developed palpitations during the pain, heart thumping in the chest
- heart beat seemed irregular and fast
- took sublingual glyceryl trinitrate spray to relieve chest pain
- cannot remember anything else until she woke up in ambulance.

Most likely diagnosis: syncopal episode due to arrhythmia secondary to ischaemic heart disease, or to postural hypotension following glyceryl trinitrate spray

Past medical history (PMH)

The past medical history can give useful information to corroborate a diagnosis or give information about the patient's general health. For example, someone presenting with chest pain who you thought might have angina could have a history of a previous pulmonary embolism, malignancy, or familial thrombophilia. Under these circumstances, although the diagnosis of angina may be correct, it would be foolish to ignore the possibility of a pulmonary embolus as the cause for the chest pain.

Two questions that would invite a patient to tell you about his or her past medical history would be:
- 'Have you had any serious illnesses in the past?' and
- 'Have you ever been admitted to hospital?'

These questions should cover major illnesses, hospital admission and operations. It is best to list replies in chronological order, for example:
- myocardial infarction 1984
- hysterectomy 1986
- pneumonia 1992
- asthma diagnosed 1994

There are also some important negatives to ask and list. In dental practice these might include:
- rheumatic fever and valvular heart disease
- asthma or chronic obstructive pulmonary disease
- epilepsy
- diabetes
- hypertension
- jaundice
- bleeding disorder

Those experienced in taking medical histories would tend to tailor important negatives according to the patient's problems. For example in a patient presenting with palpitations, cardiovascular conditions may be more important than epilepsy or jaundice.

The drug history (DH)

It is essential to record the patient's current drugs, and for students it is often helpful to note what conditions they have been prescribed for, as seen in the example below. This will teach you about the therapeutic uses of commonly prescribed drugs. In some patients with chronic conditions, such as arthritis or hypertension, it is important to list treatments that have been tried in the past but proved unsuccessful because of side effects or lack of efficacy. This avoids the relatively common problem of exposing patients to drugs that have failed them in the past.

An example of a drug history is detailed in Table 1.1. It is customary to use generic names for drugs rather than brand names, as the generic name is constant but brand names differ. If in doubt about drugs or their use consult the latest edition of the *British National Formulary* (BNF).

Allergies to drugs should also be looked for. List any positive replies giving details of the 'allergic' reaction. Sometimes patients confuse adverse reactions with allergy. For example a rash is strong evidence for an allergy, but non-specific gastrointestinal upset is a common side effect of some drugs that does not usually indicate allergy.

Table 1.1 Example of a drug history

Drug	Dose	Frequency	Condition treated
atenolol	50 mg	od (once daily)	hypertension
paracetamol	1 g	qds (four times per day)	arthritis right hip

Family history (FH)

Do any diseases 'run' in the patient's family? The family history can provide supportive evidence for a diagnosis. For example, a history of premature coronary heart disease in a first degree relative would strengthen a diagnosis of myocardial chest pain in a younger person. Other diseases that run in families include: some kidney diseases (e.g. polycystic kidneys), epilepsy, migraine, asthma and autoimmune diseases (e.g. rheumatoid arthritis).

Social history (SH)

The social history is very important as it helps you place the patient's problems in the context of their daily life. It is a vital part of the assessment of elderly patients with multiple chronic problems. Living conditions and support with personal care are useful when predicting whether the patient is likely to be able to comply with treatment once they are at home.

It is customary to ask about present, and if relevant, past occupations. For example in patients presenting with respiratory problems exposure to dust or asbestos at work would be important. Smoking habit (number of cigarettes smoked each day) and alcohol consumption (average number of units per week) are an essential part of the history as many medical and surgical conditions are linked to tobacco and alcohol use.

Systems (or symptoms) enquiry (SE)

The final part of the history is a systematic search for common symptoms that might signal medical or surgical problems. It is usual to approach this part of the history by grouping symptoms into systems such as cardiovascular, respiratory or neurological. Until you are experienced and can remember these symptoms it is best to have your own list.

Below is an example of the types of questions that may be asked, and what a positive response might mean. When a symptom is found, experienced clinicians would ask some questions around the problem in a way similar to a short history of the presenting complaint. Students often identify problems but fail to follow them up with further questions.

Cardiovascular system

Do you suffer from:
- **chest pain?** (could signal ischaemic heart disease)
- **palpitations?** (looking for abnormalities of cardiac rhythm)
- **high blood pressure?** (a risk factor for cardiac and cerebrovascular disease)
- **shortness of breath when lying down in bed?** (orthopnoea due to pulmonary venous congestion. Occurs in heart failure – but remember that some patients with airways obstruction also get short of breath when lying flat!)
- **waking in the middle of the night short of breath?** (paroxysmal nocturnal dyspnoea (PND) in heart failure due to the development of pulmonary oedema)
- **shortness of breath on exertion?** (abbreviated to SOBOE in case notes, a symptom of cardiac or respiratory disease)
- **fatigue?** (a common symptom of chronic and severe cardiac or respiratory disease)
- **pain in the back of your calves when walking?** (intermittent claudication due to peripheral vascular disease)

Respiratory system

Do you suffer from
- **wheezing?** (episodic wheezing is the hallmark of asthma)
- **shortness of breath?** (may be more relevant here if no cardiac symptoms but plenty of respiratory ones!)
- **chest pain which is worse on inspiration?** (pleuritic chest pain due to inflammation of the pleura due to infection or infarction. May also be present in musculoskeletal chest pain)
- **cough?** (a common feature of respiratory infection or malignancy)
- **do you cough up phlegm (or sputum)?** (record amount and colour, e.g. longstanding sputum production of large volumes occasionally blood stained would be consistent with bronchiectasis. Rusty coloured sputum – a mixture of pus and blood – is common in pneumococcal pneumonia)
- **do you cough up blood?** (haemoptysis – should alert you to the possibility of carcinoma of the lung, tuberculosis, or with the right history pulmonary embolus)

Gastrointestinal tract

Do you suffer from:
- **weight loss?** (non-specific sign of poor nutrition due to illness, rapid weight loss is a good marker of the severity of illness)

- **difficulty swallowing?** (dysphagia – may signal a stricture of the oesophagus due to malignancy or inflammation)
- **anorexia and vomiting?** (may occur in carcinoma of the stomach and in peptic ulcer disease. Vomiting blood is called haematemesis)
- **abdominal pain?** (the site of the pain can locate the likely area of disease e.g. epigastric – pancreas or stomach, lower abdominal – colon or bladder)
- **have you had a change in bowel habit?** (define the normal habit for the patient, e.g. once daily, and then ask about diarrhoea, constipation and the presence of mucus slime or blood in the motion. The last three together may signal inflammatory bowel disease. Constipations and blood may be due to carcinoma of the colon or rectum)
- **black motions?** (melaena is due to altered blood in the motion from an upper gastrointestinal bleed or iron tablets!)

Genitourinary system

Do you suffer from:
- **dysuria?** (pain when passing urine – a sign of infection or stricture)
- **passing blood in the urine?** (haematuria – a feature of infection and malignancy)
- **getting up at night to pass urine?** (Nocturia can be present in prostatism [see below], diabetes, hypercalcaemia, or infection)
- **vaginal discharge?** (due to infection)
- **vaginal bleeding** after the menopause? (post menopausal bleeding [PMB]) or in younger women bleeding between periods? (intermenstrual bleeding [IMB]) (both can signal malignancy)

In men **prostatism** describes symptoms due to bladder outflow obstruction caused by an enlarged prostate from benign prostatic hyperplasia or malignancy. Symptoms include **a poor stream**, **hesitancy**, **nocturia**, and **terminal dribbling** (urine continues to flow after the patient thinks he has stopped)

Nervous system

Do you suffer from:
- **weakness or numbness of an arm or leg?** (focal weakness or numbness may indicate cerebrovascular disease)
- **pins and needles?** (a non-specific symptom that is commonly reported by many normal patients, but when marked it can signal peripheral neuropathy)
- **visual disturbance?** (double vision – diplopia – may indicate a new ocular palsy, other disturbances like fortification spectra – zigzag lines and bright shapes – are reported in migraine)

- **headache?** (the differential diagnosis of headaches is an important topic for a dental student. For example being able to distinguish dental pain from facial pain due to earache, inflamed sinuses, trigeminal neuralgia, migraine, and headache due to meningitis and brain tumours)
- **poor co-ordination and balance?** (this can occur in diseases of the cerebellum and inner ear, or by involvement of nerve tracts such as peripheral nerves or those connecting the cerebellum to the inner ear)

Skin and joints

Do you suffer from
- **skin rashes?** (rashes can be due to primary skin diseases; drug, food or contact allergy; or as a manifestation of a systemic disease. When present record the site, duration of illness, and factors that may be involved)
- **joint pains?** (it is important to try to distinguish between four common forms of chronic arthritis – osteoarthritis, rheumatoid arthritis, gout and psoriatic arthropathy. Define which joints are affected, whether there is early morning stiffness, and swelling or deformity of joints – the latter can be looked for during the examination of the patient. It is essential for dental students to recognise the possibility of severe rheumatoid arthritis that might signal subluxation of the atlantoaxial joint in the neck. In these patients injudicious extension of the neck in the dental chair may result in severe cervical cord damage!)

At the end of the history

At the end of the history you should have a very good idea of the patient's presenting complaints, the time course of these symptoms and how these relate to the past medical history. Good clinicians would usually have a definite working diagnosis by this stage, looking to confirm their suspicions during the clinical examination and by further tests.

As a dental student you should also be thinking of the patient's present and past medical history in the context of any planned dental work, trying to predict problems that might arise in the dental chair.

Further reading

Ford, M.J., Munro, J.F. (2000) *Introduction to Clinical Examination.* 7th edition. Edinburgh, Churchill Livingstone.

Websites

Merck Manual of Medical Information:
    http://www.merckhomeedition.com/
Cancer Web: http://cancerweb.ncl.ac.uk/omd/

CHAPTER 2
Clinical Examination

Examination is performed once a history has been taken. In this chapter, sufficient detail will be given of the methods of clinical examination to allow a dentist to assess his or her patient prior to dental treatment or if an emergency arises. The details given are focused on the needs of the dentist and it is not intended to provide a comprehensive disclosure of methods that would be appropriate for a medical graduate.

In most cases the dentist will expect to examine their patient in a dental chair or perhaps on the floor if an emergency arises. The dentist will usually be faced with a clothed patient rather than one who has undressed especially for examination, although it may be appropriate for the dentist to loosen the patient's clothes for part of the examination. Some details of examination will be presented in more detail than is actually required, to offer a better understanding of points of theory.

Basic principles

Every patient has the right to privacy and comfort during the examination. This may mean screening off an area if others can observe the examination. If it is the first time you have met the patient you should introduce yourself. It is usual to examine a patient from their right side if you are right handed and from their left side if you are left handed. Take care not to cause the patient any discomfort, especially if they have any areas of the body that might be tender. If a patient is short of breath they are often more comfortable sitting up. A male dentist examining a female patient may need a chaperone. On completion of the examination, the details should be recorded in a systematic fashion.

General examination

Demeanour

On first meeting the patient you will already have noticed their general demeanour. Your observations of their body build, posture, gait, behaviour and speech will already have told you if they are overweight or thin, bent over by arthritis, aggressive or suffering from a neurological problem that has impaired their speech. If a patient appears hot and sweaty they may be pyrexial and their temperature should be taken (the normal body temperature is 37°C).

Colour

The patient may have a bluish tinge to the lips and tongue, indicating central cyanosis due to an elevated blood level of desaturated haemoglobin, or to the fingers, suggesting peripheral cyanosis due to excessive extraction of oxygen from the blood perhaps associated with sluggish blood flow.

Anaemia is suggested by pallor – best appreciated by examining the conjunctivae or buccal mucosa.

A high degree of red colour of the face (plethoric facies) is seen when the patient's haemoglobin is too high, as in polycythaemia.

Jaundice is suggested by a yellow discoloration of the sclera of the eye and is due to an excess of liver-derived bilirubin in the blood.

Other colour changes may be apparent such as white patches on the hands or face (vitiligo), increased melanin pigmentation on the buccal mucosa (as in Addison's disease) or facial pigmentation, e.g. as a consequence of the patient taking the drug amiodarone.

The hands

The hands are readily available for inspection and can give a lot of useful information. The colour of the fingers may be blue indicating Raynaud's phenomenon (blood vessels vasoconstricting too easily to the cold) or peripheral cyanosis. The nails may be pale (as in anaemia), there could be redness of the palms or 'spider naevi' (telangiectasia, see Colour Plate 13) due to vasodilation as a consequence of circulating oestrogens in liver disease, and the palmar creases might show the pigmentation of Addison's disease.

The joints of the fingers may show the changes of arthritis with swelling of the proximal interphalangeal joints, as seen in rheumatoid

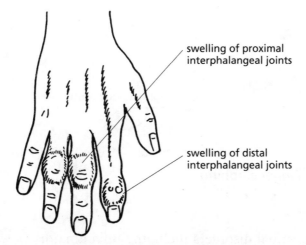

swelling of proximal
interphalangeal joints

swelling of distal
interphalangeal joints

Figure 2.1 Joints of the hand in rheumatoid arthritis.

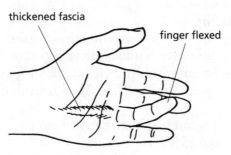

thickened fascia

finger flexed

Figure 2.2 Dupuytren's contracture.

arthritis (Figure 2.1), or of the distal interphalangeal joints, as in osteoarthritis (when so-called Heberden's nodes are also seen as nodular swellings around the joint). The fingers themselves are tapered with a waxy thickened skin in the connective tissue disorder scleroderma, and the whole hand can be enlarged in a 'spade-like' manner in the pituitary condition called acromegaly. Dupuytren's contracture, a condition of thickening of the palmar fascia (Figure 2.2), is easily recognised: it is associated with liver disease and anticonvulsant therapy.

The nails require special attention. Finger clubbing (see Colour Plate 4) denotes a bulbous swelling of the terminal phalanges with loss of the normal angle between the nail fold and the nail (Figure 2.3). Finger clubbing can be a sign of:
• serious heart disease, e.g. a cyanotic congenital anomaly or infective endocarditis
• lung disease, e.g. carcinoma of the bronchus, bronchiectasis, or fibrosing alveolitis

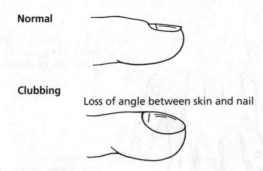

Figure 2.3 Finger clubbing.

• gastrointestinal disorders including inflammatory bowel disease and cirrhosis
• or it can be a congenital occurrence in its own right.

The nails may also show the features of psoriasis, i.e. separation of the nail from the nail bed ('onycholysis', see Colour Plate 1) and nail pitting, the splinter haemorrhages (see Colour Plate 8) characteristic of infective endocarditis, or telangiectasia at the nail folds – as seen in vasculitis (Figure 2.4). The 'spoon-shaped' nail (koilonychia, see Colour Plate 3) of iron deficiency is easily recognised.

Tremor of the outstretched hand can indicate:
• an overactive thyroid (thyrotoxicosis)
• carbon dioxide retention of chronic obstructive lung disease
• beta agonist therapy (e.g. salbutamol) for asthma
• liver disease
• anxiety

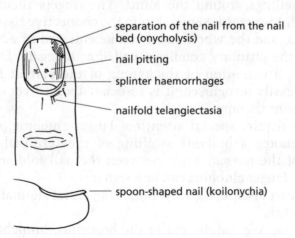

Figure 2.4 Nail abnormalities.

- or, in the case of the 'pill-rolling' tremor seen at rest, Parkinson's disease.

Sweaty palms may signify thyrotoxicosis.

The face and skull

Examination of the face will include shape and symmetry, lumps and skin colour, expression and speech, and external inspection of the eyes and ears. Any asymmetry or hyperplasia of the skull or facial bones should be noted (causes include fibrous dysplasia, Paget's disease and condylar hyperplasia). Dentists would not expect to perform ophthalmoscopy or to look inside the ears. An oral examination is a routine dental procedure and will not be covered here.

An asymmetrical face may be due to drooping of one side of the mouth, as seen in facial (seventh cranial) nerve palsy (Bell's palsy, Figure 2.5, Colour Plate 23) when the eyelid can droop, but facial asymmetry also might be the result of a stroke. A drooping eyelid (ptosis) with a dilated pupil and an eye that looks downwards and outwards can signify a palsy of the third cranial nerve.

The expression of the face is immobile in Parkinson's disease (and sometimes too in depression or Alzheimer's disease) and startled in thyrotoxicosis (due to prominence of the eyes, exophthalmos [see Colour Plate 21], and the white of the sclera being visible all around the pupil). In Down's syndrome, the head is small, the face flat, the node short and squat, and the eyes show slanting palpebral fissures and an epicanthic fold (a skin fold on the upper eyelid that covers the inner corner of the eye).

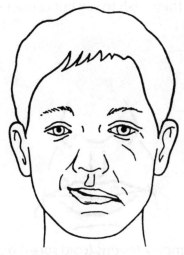

Figure 2.5 Facial nerve (Bell's) palsy.

Swelling of the sides of the face may be due to enlargement of the parotid glands, as seen for example in mumps, when there is tenderness, or in the granulomatous condition, sarcoidosis, when the swelling is painless.

Inspection of the eyes will reveal jaundice or exophthalmos, or an abnormality of the pupils. A unilateral small pupil, in association with ptosis on the same side suggests a lesion of the cervical sympathetic nerves (Horner's syndrome). An acutely red eye may indicate an adenovirus infection but more serious causes need to be considered (see Colour Plate 39 and Chapter 12, Ophthalmological Diseases).

External examination of the ears might demonstrate a dermatitis of the ear or a tumour such as a basal cell carcinoma.

A skin examination of the face may reveal:
- a common rash such as an eczema (see Colour Plate 41) or acne
- infective lesions such as bacterial boils or cold sores (herpes simplex, Figure 2.6, see also Colour Plate 29) (which are important to recognise in dentistry because of their infectious potential)
- benign growths (e.g. viral warts, see Colour Plate 27)
- malignant tumours (e.g. basal cell carcinoma or malignant melanoma, see Colour Plate 47) that need to be notified to the patient's medical doctor.

Speech is affected in several neurological conditions including cerebrovascular disease, multiple sclerosis and motor neuron disease. The patient's speech may be normal in language but slurred with poor articulation (dysarthria) due to cerebellar disease or a disorder of the motor neurons. The voice may be hoarse in disorders of the vocal cord or in neuromuscular weakness (dysphonia). When there is impairment of use of language and the patient may understand what is said or what they wish to say but cannot say it, the condition is termed 'dysphasia'.

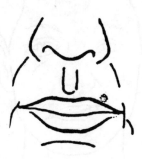

Figure 2.6 Herpes simplex lesions (cold sores) occur on the lips.

The neck

Swellings in the neck can be from lymph nodes, the thyroid gland, salivary glands or occasionally from other causes. The first step in examination of the neck is to inspect from the front. Look for asymmetry, and to see if the swelling moves on swallowing – a sign of a thyroid swelling as the thyroid is attached to the larynx by the pretracheal fascia – or if it is pulsatile (suggesting it might be an arterial mass).

Palpation of the neck is usually undertaken from behind. For enlarged lymph nodes, feel under the mandible, over the anterior and posterior triangles of the neck, and along the top and beneath the clavicles (Figure 2.7). Lymphadenopathy may be due to malignant disease, e.g. a lymphoma or an oral squamous cell carcinoma, or to an infection, e.g. glandular fever (infectious mononucleosis) or German measles (rubella).

Swelling of the salivary glands (see Colour Plate 38) can result from duct obstruction, bacterial infection, systemic infection (e.g. mumps), sarcoidosis, Sjogren's syndrome or neoplasia.

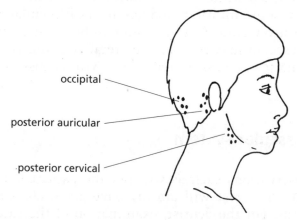

occipital

posterior auricular

posterior cervical

Figure 2.7a Enlarged lymph nodes (lymphadenopathy) side view.

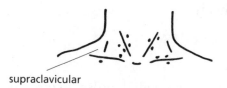

supraclavicular

also consider toxoplasmosis
salivary gland swelling may be caused by mumps (painful)

Figure 2.7b Enlarged lymph nodes (lymphadenopathy) front view.

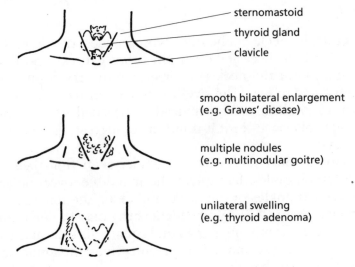

sternomastoid

thyroid gland

clavicle

smooth bilateral enlargement
(e.g. Graves' disease)

multiple nodules
(e.g. multinodular goitre)

unilateral swelling
(e.g. thyroid adenoma)

Figure 2.8 Thyroid gland.

Palpation of the anterior neck for a swollen thyroid (goitre) is usually performed while the patient swallows a sip of water. The thyroid may show multiple nodules in multinodular goitre (Figure 2.8, see also Colour Plate 19), smooth bilateral enlargement in Graves' disease, or may reveal a unilateral swelling as in a thyroid adenoma (that can be associated with thyrotoxicosis) or a thyroid carcinoma.

Cardiovascular system

General observations such as whether the patient is cyanosed or short of breath at rest will already have given clues about their cardiac status. For the dentist, examination of the cardiovascular system will include the pulse, blood pressure and overt signs of cardiac failure (e.g. an elevated jugular venous pressure or peripheral oedema), with only a brief mention of palpation of the chest and auscultation of the heart.

The pulse

It is usual to examine the radial pulse using the tips of one's index and middle fingers pressed lightly onto the patient's wrist (Figure 2.9). An assessment of the rate, rhythm and character of the pulse is possible. The pulse rate is measured by counting the number of beats over a timed period of say, 30 seconds. The normal pulse

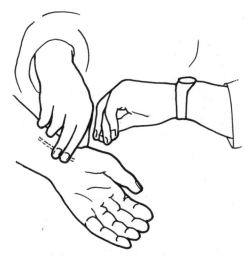

Figure 2.9 Taking the pulse.

rate is 72 beats per minute. Bradycardia is defined as less than 60 beats per minute and tachycardia as more than 100. Bradycardia is commonly due to beta blocking drugs but may be seen in trained athletes or with certain types of heart block. Tachycardia is due to various types of dysrhythmias (see Chapter 3, Cardiovascular Diseases) but might just be a sign of anxiety.

The rhythm of the pulse should be assessed as either regular (although frequently in young patients it quickens with inspiration and hence is called sinus arrhythmia) or irregular, in which case it may be chaotically irregular, as in atrial fibrillation. It is difficult for inexperienced observers to easily define the character of the pulse but the collapsing pulse found in aortic incompetence, characterised by a more sudden rise in the wave form than normal (felt as a 'slapping' against the palpating fingers), can be appreciated.

Blood pressure

When the blood pressure is measured the systolic and diastolic pressures within the brachial artery are recorded. The patient should be comfortable and lying or sitting. A blood pressure cuff of 12 cm width is usually used but a larger one may be needed for obese patients. The cuff is placed over the upper arm over the brachial artery after any tight-fitting garments have been removed or loosened (Figure 2.10). While palpating the radial artery, the sphygmomanometer cuff is inflated to just above the systolic pressure, denoted by obliteration of the radial pulse. The stethoscope is then applied to the area of the brachial artery at the antecubital

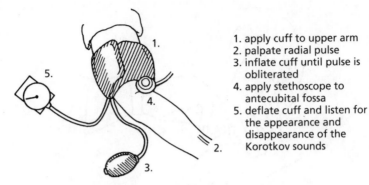

1. apply cuff to upper arm
2. palpate radial pulse
3. inflate cuff until pulse is obliterated
4. apply stethoscope to antecubital fossa
5. deflate cuff and listen for the appearance and disappearance of the Korotkov sounds

Figure 2.10 Taking the blood pressure.

fossa and the cuff is slowly deflated. The systolic pressure is recorded as soon as the 'Korotkov' sounds of the pulse beat are audible; the diastolic pressure is marked by the disappearance of these sounds. The blood pressure is recorded as millimetres of mercury (mm Hg). The normal is 120/80. Hypertension is discussed in Chapter 3, Cardiovascular Diseases.

Signs of cardiac failure

A patient with heart failure may be short of breath at rest, uncomfortable lying down and have a resting tachycardia. The jugular venous pressure may be elevated, the ankles may be swollen due to peripheral oedema and crepitations may be heard on auscultation of the lungs.

The jugular venous pressure (JVP) gives an indication of the blood pressure in the right side of the heart. It is measured by positioning the patient at 45 degrees with their head turned to the left, and observing for pulsation of the internal jugular vein deep to the sternomastoid muscle (Figure 2.11).

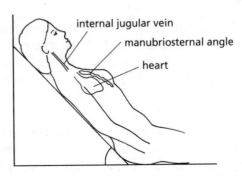

internal jugular vein
manubriosternal angle
heart

Figure 2.11 Measuring jugular venous pressure (JVP).

Pulsations of the carotid artery can be easily mistaken for the internal jugular vein but are readily palpable and do not alter with respiration or light compression of the abdomen, both of which elevate the JVP. Light compression of the vein just above the clavicle obliterates the JVP. The JVP is measured as the height (in cms) of the top of the pulse wave above the manubriosternal angle. The normal JVP is less than 3 cm. Elevation suggests right heart failure.

Oedema is due to fluid overload and when of cardiac origin is accompanied by an elevated JVP. In the ambulant patient, oedema is seen first at the ankles, where firm pressure with a finger for five seconds will leave an indentation ('pitting oedema'). In a patient confined to bed, the oedema can be seen at the sacral area. Generalised oedema can also result from a low serum albumin, e.g. as a result of kidney or liver disease. Oedema of the lower legs can be secondary to venous disease.

Palpation and auscultation

Examination of the heart itself begins with palpation of the precordium, laying the palm of the right hand over the left side of the chest to feel for the most lateral and downward impulse of the heart – the 'apex beat'. This is usually located at the mid-clavicular line in the fifth intercostal space. In cardiac failure, the apex beat may be displaced laterally if the heart is enlarged.

The precordium is also palpated for heart murmurs which, if loud, can be felt as a vibration (a 'thrill'). Auscultation of the heart with a stethoscope is normally performed using the diaphragm side of the instrument. Apply this first on to the area of the apex beat and then over other parts of the anterior chest to listen for the heart sounds and for murmurs from the heart valves.

The first heart sound is mainly due to closure of the mitral valve; the second is caused by closure of the aortic and pulmonary valves. A third heart sound may be audible in cardiac failure. Stenosis or incompetence of the different heart valves produce specific murmurs (Figure 2.12).

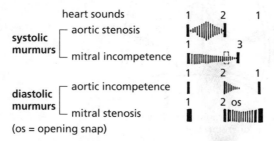

Figure 2.12 Heart murmurs.

Respiratory system

Some general features of respiratory disease such as shortness of breath, cyanosis or finger clubbing will already be evident. For the dentist, examination of the chest mainly consists of inspection and palpation; only brief details of percussion and auscultation will be given.

Inspection

Assess whether the chest is normally shaped and symmetrical. In most people the anterior–posterior diameter is less than the transverse but in chronic obstructive airways disease the chest overexpands and the cross section of the thorax becomes rounder (i.e. 'barrel-chested', see Colour Plate 9). Normal breathing is done using the diaphragm which goes down on inspiration (Figure 2.13). Observe the patient's breathing:
• Do both sides of the chest expand on inspiration? (asymmetrical expansion suggests an obstructed bronchus).
• Is inspiration longer than expiration? (as is normally the case) or is expiration prolonged? (as in asthma).
• Is inspiration curtailed by pain? (e.g. due to pleurisy from a chest infection or a pulmonary embolus).
• Is there an audible wheeze? (to suggest bronchospasm).
• Does the patient breath out using pursed lips to prevent collapse of the bronchial walls? (a feature of obstructive airways disease).
• Count the respiratory rate: the normal is 14 breaths per minute. More may signify respiratory disease.

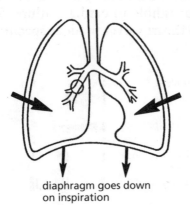

indrawing of the intercostal spaces on inspiration indicates bronchoconstriction

diaphragm goes down on inspiration

Figure 2.13 Normal respiration.

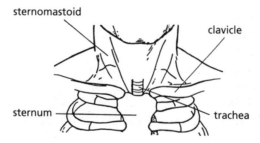

Figure 2.14 Location of the trachea.

Palpation

The trachea is normally in the midline of the neck, equidistant between the sternomastoid muscles and in the middle of the suprasternal notch (Figure 2.14). Deviation to one side or the other can indicate a collapsed lung, a large pleural effusion (fluid in the pleural space), or a pneumothorax (air in the pleural space due to a hole in the lung).

To assess the trachea, place the tip of the index finger in the suprasternal notch. If the fingertip fits more easily on one side or the other, the trachea may be deviated. Palpation can be used to measure inspiration. Place both hands fingers outermost across the front of the chest, with the thumbs just touching in the midline. Hold the fingertips closely to the chest and let the thumbs move towards and away from each other, thus demonstrating the range of respiratory movements.

Percussion and auscultation

The lungs and hence the thorax contain air and when percussed will produce an audible note. If air is not present beneath the area of the chest that is percussed, e.g. because of pleural fluid around the lung or thickening in the lung, the resonance of the note will be dull. Conversely, if there is a large air-filled space, e.g. with a pneumo-thorax, the note will be hyper-resonant.

To percuss the chest, place the left middle finger on the chest and strike sharply on its middle phalanx using the tip of the flexed middle finger of the right hand, with the movement coming from the wrist. Percuss the thorax from top to bottom, anteriorly and posteriorly, comparing the right with the left as it is done.

To auscultate, apply the diaphragm of the stethoscope to the chest wall and listen as the patient breathes in and out gently through an open mouth. Breath sounds are generated by vibrations of the vocal cords that resonate down the bronchial tree until conducted to the chest wall. The intensity of breath sounds increases during inspiration and fades in expiration.

Examine all areas of the chest. Breath sounds may be reduced by a pleural effusion or increased by lung thickening. Sounds of wheeze (rhonchi), signifying bronchospasm, or crackles (crepitations) from secretions in the bronchial tree (suggesting infection or heart failure), may be added.

The abdomen

It is unlikely that a dentist will be called on to examine the abdomen unless a patient presents suddenly and incidentally with severe abdominal pain. The basic principles are as for other systems and consist of inspection and palpation (sometimes with percussion and auscultation). Any obvious masses, distension, pulsation, asymmetry or colour change in the skin will be seen on observation. Palpation of the abdomen is mostly done using the right hand which is gently applied to the abdominal wall, starting at an area away from the site of any pain. There are specific methods for the palpation of the liver, spleen and kidneys but these are outside the remit of this chapter. Palpation allows the identification of any masses, enlargement of the liver, spleen or kidneys, and permits the location of areas of tenderness and rigidity of the abdominal muscles (which can indicate underlying inflammation).

Nervous system

The dentist will form a general impression of the patient's mental state, intellect and ability to communicate on first meeting them and after a brief consultation. It would not be expected that a dentist would need to perform a full neurological assessment of the cranial nerves, muscle power, tendon reflexes, sensation and co-ordination. However, it may be relevant to examine the function of certain cranial nerves and familiarity with the Glasgow Coma Scale (see Table 2.1) is useful if a patient collapses unconscious.

Cranial nerves V, VII and XII

The fifth cranial nerve (trigeminal) has sensory and motor components. The sensory part supplies the face, scalp, tongue and buccal mucosa (including the corneal reflex); the motor innervates the

Table 2.1 The Glasgow Coma Scale
(E+M+V= 3 minimum, 15 maximum)

Assessment	Score
Eye opening (E)	
spontaneous	4
to speech	3
to pain	2
nil	1
Best motor response (m)	
obeys	6
localises	5
withdraws	4
abnormal flexion	3
extensor response	2
nil	1
Verbal response (v)	
orientated	5
confused conversation	4
inappropriate words	3
incomprehensible sounds	2
nil	1

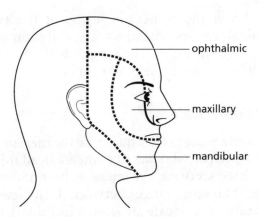

Figure 2.15 Sensory divisions of the fifth cranial nerve (trigeminal).

muscles of mastication and the jaw jerk (Figure 2.15). The three sensory divisions of the trigeminal nerve, the mandibular, maxillary and ophthalmic, are tested on each side using a piece of cotton wool for light touch and a paperclip for pain. The corneal reflex is assessed by gently touching the cornea from the side with a wisp of cotton wool, provoking a blinking reflex if intact. The cranial nerves are discussed in Chapter 8, Neurological Diseases.

Motor function is assessed by asking the patient to open the mouth against resistance (the jaw deviates to the side of any weakness of the pterygoid muscles), by palpating the masseter muscles with the jaw clenched and, for the jaw jerk, by asking the patient to let their mouth hang loosely open, placing the examiner's thumb on the chin and striking it lightly with a tendon hammer.

The seventh cranial nerve (facial) supplies taste sensation to the anterior two-thirds of the tongue and innervates the muscles of facial expression. The motor innervation of the upper parts of the face comes from both sides of the motor cortex with the consequence that a unilateral upper motor neuron lesion affects muscle movements of the lower face more than those of the forehead. A lower motor neuron lesion affects upper and lower facial muscle function equally.

Inspection can show a lack of wrinkling of the forehead or drooping of one side of the mouth (see Colour Plate 23). The upper facial muscles can be assessed by asking the patient to wrinkle their forehead or tightly screw their eyes up. The lower facial muscles are tested by asking the patient to blow out their cheeks and also to grimace and show their teeth. The taste sensations of sweet, bitter, sour and salt can be evaluated by applying small amounts of sugar, quinine, vinegar and salt on to the anterior tongue on orange sticks.

A unilateral lower motor neuron lesion of the twelfth cranial nerve (hypoglossal) causes weakness, fasciculation and atrophy of the ipsilateral tongue muscles. The tongue deviates towards the side of weakness when protruded (see Colour Plate 24).

The Glasgow Coma Scale

The Glasgow Coma Scale gives a quantitative measure of the neurological state of a patient who has sustained a head injury. The scale is divided into three sections: eye opening, best motor response and verbal response. The score ranges between 3 (the least) and 15 (the maximum). Details of the scale are shown in Table 2.1.

Further reading

Ford, M.J., Munro, J.F. (2000) *Introduction to Clinical Examination*. 7th edition. Edinburgh, Churchill Livingstone.

Websites

Physical exam study guides:
  http://medinfo.ufl.edu/year1/bcs/clist/index.html
The Visible Human Project:
  http://www.nlm.nih.gov/research/visible/visible_human.html
Heart sounds:
  http://www.bcm.tmc.edu/class2000/sims/HeartSounds.html
Lung sounds:
  http://www.muhealth.org/~shrp/rtwww/rcweb/docs/sounds.html
Photo rounds: http://www.mdchoice.com/photo/photos.asp

SECTION 2
Diseases and Conditions

CHAPTER 3
Cardiovascular Diseases

Dentists see many patients with ischaemic, congenital and valvular heart disease and need to know how to manage these cases safely, what the significance of any medication may be (e.g. the potential for drug interaction or side effects from treatment), and what to do if a patient develops acute symptoms during dental treatment.

Ischaemic heart disease

Iftikhar U. Haq

Ischaemic heart disease is a result of an imbalance between myocardial oxygen supply and demand. The commonest underlying pathology is atherosclerosis of coronary arteries (Figure 3.1). Patients with coronary ischaemia complain of angina or may suffer a myocardial infarction. Fixed risk factors include increasing age, male sex, positive family history, and race (higher in British Asians). The major modifiable risk factors are cigarette smoking, hyper-lipidaemia, hypertension, and diabetes mellitus. Poor oral health, e.g. the presence of dental caries, is thought by some investigators to be associated with ischaemic heart disease.

Symptoms and investigations

Angina is typically described as a crushing, tight or squeezing pain. It is most commonly retrosternal and may radiate to the sides of the chest, down the left arm or less commonly right arm, up to the neck and jaw, or occasionally to the epigastrium or back. It may be associated with shortness of breath. Angina typically lasts for minutes and is relieved by rest. Clamminess, nausea, vomiting and sweating are features of myocardial infarction.

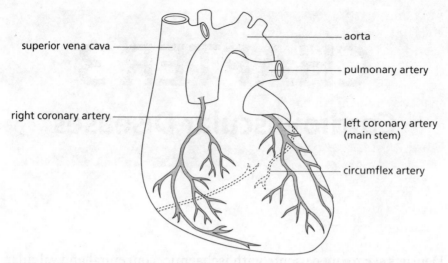

superior vena cava

aorta

pulmonary artery

right coronary artery

left coronary artery
(main stem)

circumflex artery

Figure 3.1 The right and left coronary arteries come off from the ascending aorta.

The electrocardiograph (ECG: a recording of the electrical activity of the heart) during an attack commonly shows ST segment depression or T wave inversion. The exercise ECG is an indicator of exercise performance. Nuclear imaging is used to assess myocardial structure and function. Coronary angiography visualises the coronary arteries radiographically, using a contrast dye that is injected into the vessels.

Unstable angina is a manifestation of coronary ischaemia characterised by chest pain, sometimes of increasing intensity and present for days, which is present at rest or on mild exertion in the absence of elevation of the ST segment (as seen in acute myocardial infarction) on the ECG. It is a medical emergency since it may lead to acute myocardial infarction, and urgent referral is needed.

Treatment

Non-coronary causes for angina should be sought and treated appropriately, for example valvular heart disease, intermittent tachycardias, hyperthyroidism or anaemia. Risk factors should be evaluated, and steps should be taken to correct them.

All patients should be prescribed aspirin 75–300 mg daily, as this lowers the incidence of subsequent myocardial infarction and death. If cholesterol is >5.0 mmol/l after diet, patients also benefit from statins to lower cholesterol. During an acute attack, the patient should stop any precipitating factors such as exercise, and take sublingual glyceryl trinitrate (GTN). Patients may take sublingual GTN prophylactically before exertion.

When angina occurs frequently, regular prophylactic therapy is given, e.g. beta adrenoreceptor blockers, nitrates, calcium antagonists, and potassium channel openers.

Angioplasty, in which a small balloon is inflated in the coronary artery, can relieve an obstruction. Surgery is considered in patients whose symptoms persist despite optimal medical management.

Summary: Ischaemic heart disease

- **Cause**: a common cause is atherosclerosis of the coronary arteries.
- **Risk factors** include family history, hyperlipidaemia, cigarette smoking, hypertension and diabetes.
- **Pathophysiology**: It is the result of an imbalance between the myocardial oxygen supply and the myocardial oxygen demand.
- **Angina** is a common symptom in which there is a crushing or tight pain retrosternally or down the left arm.
- **Acute myocardial infarction** occurs when the coronary artery blood supply to cardiac muscle is occluded. It is characterised by chest pain with clamminess, nausea and sweating.
- **Treatment** of ischaemic heart disease includes aspirin (reduces incidence of myocardial infarction), a statin (if there is hyper-lipidaemia), GTN (for angina attack), and prophylactic measures such as beta blockers or other drugs. Severe cases are treated with angioplasty or surgery. Myocardial infarction is treated in specialised acute medical units according to strict protocols.

Myocardial infarction

Iftikhar U. Haq

Myocardial infarction (MI) affects 5 people per 1000 per year in the UK, and is the most common cause of death in the Western world. The overall fatality in the first month is 50%, and about one half of these deaths occur within the first two hours. The in-hospital mortality is 20%.

Diagnosis

The diagnosis is based on the history, ECG and enzyme changes. Cardiac enzymes are intracellular enzymes that leak out of infarcted myocardium into the bloodstream. Troponin is the first enzyme to be released followed by creatinine kinase, aspartate amino-transferase, and lactic dehydrogenase. An ECG will show elevation of the ST segment.

Management

The aim is to prevent or treat cardiac arrest and to relieve pain. The patient should be managed in a coronary care unit. Intravenous opioids such as diamorphine are given for pain relief with high dose oxygen. Patients seen within 12 hours of the onset of pain are given thrombolysis. Aspirin 300 mg should be prescribed early. Beta blockers intravenously in the acute phase limit infarct size.

Complications

Complications include sudden death, arrhythmias, persistent pain, cardiac failure, mitral incompetence, pericarditis, cardiac rupture and ventricular septal defects, mural thrombus, ventricular aneurysm and pulmonary emboli. Routine dental surgery should be delayed for three months following an acute myocardial infarction.

Summary: Myocardial infarction

• **Definition**: partial or complete blockage of a coronary artery that can result in chest or arm pain, heart failure, cardiac arrest, arrhythmia, and death.
• **Diagnosis**: based on history, findings, ECG changes and changes in cardiac enzyme levels.
• **Management**: admit to coronary care unit; prevent cardiac arrest, relieve pain and limit infarct size.

Heart failure

Iftikhar U. Haq

Heart failure occurs when the heart is unable to maintain sufficient cardiac output to meet the demands of the body, despite normal filling pressures (Figure 3.2). The incidence rises with age, and is present in 1% of the over 65s. The mortality in severe heart failure is about 50% at one year. Common causes include myocardial ischaemia and infarction, hypertension, valvular heart disease, drugs, e.g. some anti-arrhythmics, arrhythmias, e.g. atrial fibrillation, and cardiomyopathy.

Clinical features

Left heart failure is characterised by exertional dyspnoea, ortho-pnoea, paroxysmal nocturnal dyspnoea, fatigue, wheeze, cough, and

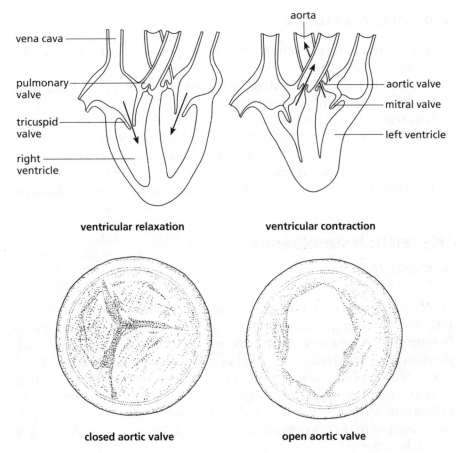

ventricular relaxation   **ventricular contraction**

closed aortic valve   **open aortic valve**

This diagram shows the position of the heart valves and the direction of blood flow during ventricular filling (left) and contraction (right) with the corresponding state of the aortic valve (i.e. closed and open).

Figure 3.2 Cardiac output is dependent on ventricular contraction.

haemoptysis. Right heart failure may occur secondary to chronic lung disease. It is commonly secondary to left ventricular failure, in which case the term congestive cardiac failure is used. Symptoms include fatigue, nausea, wasting, swollen ankles, abdominal discomfort, anorexia and breathlessness.

Treatment

Diuretics relieve the symptoms of heart failure and angiotensin converting enzyme (ACE) inhibitors improve symptoms and prognosis. An oral nitrate and hydralazine, an angiotensin II receptor antagonist, digoxin, spironolactone and beta blockers may be used. For patients with severe heart failure, heart transplantation should be considered.

Summary: Heart failure

- **Heart failure occurs** when cardiac output is insufficient for the demands of the body.
- **Causes** include myocardial ischaemia, valvular heart disease, arrhythmias and cardiomyopathy.
- **Features**: left ventricular failure is characterised by shortness of breath, cough and fatigue. Right ventricular failure is often found with left heart failure (i.e. 'congestive cardiac failure') and is characterised by swollen ankles, breathlessness and fatigue.
- **Treatment** is with diuretics, ACE inhibitors, nitrates and digoxin.

Hypercholesterolaemia

Iftikhar U. Haq

Hypercholesterolaemia is prevalent in Western societies. In the UK, over 50% of people over 45 years have total cholesterol above 6.5 mmol/l. Coronary heart disease (CHD) risk increases with increasing concentrations of total and low density lipoprotein (LDL) cholesterol, and decreases with increasing concentrations of high density lipoprotein (HDL) cholesterol. However, cholesterol concentration by itself is of limited value and of more importance is to assess the patient's overall coronary risk, of which cholesterol is one risk factor.

Causes of secondary hyperlipidaemia should be treated. These include diabetes mellitus, excess alcohol, hypothyroidism, cholestasis, chronic renal impairment, nephrotic syndrome and oestrogens. Patients with evidence of atherosclerotic vascular disease should be treated with 'statins', which inhibit the enzyme HMG-CoA reductase and reduce concentrations of total and LDL cholesterol. This class of drugs has been shown to reduce mortality in this group of patients.

For people without overt vascular disease, CHD risk should be estimated using tables (such as those found in the *British National Formulary*). Current guidelines suggest treating people with statins if estimated risk of CHD events is greater than 30% over 10 years.

Summary: hypercholesterolaemia

- **Prevalence**: >50% of people over 45 years in the UK.
- **Risk factor**: a high blood cholesterol increases chance of ischaemic heart disease.
- **Treatment**: diet, 'statins'.

Congenital heart disease

Iftikhar U. Haq

Patients with congenital heart disease usually require prophylactic antibiotics prior to dental procedures. The most important congenital heart defects are listed here.

Ventricular septal defect

Ventricular septal defect (VSD) is the most common congenital heart lesion accounting for about one third of all malformations. Blood moves from the high pressure left ventricle to the right ventricle. The left ventricle may be hypertrophic. If the defect is large, pulmonary flow increases leading to obliterative pulmonary vascular changes. Symptoms include dyspnoea and fatigue but may be absent. Antibiotic prophylaxis is advised to prevent endocarditis. Significant defects should be closed surgically to prevent pulmonary hypertension.

Atrial septal defect

Atrial septal defect (ASD) accounts for 10% of congenital heart defects. The communication between the atria allows for left to right atrial shunting. Atrial arryhthmias are common. There may be increased right heart output giving a heart murmur. Most patients are asymptomatic. A few have dyspnoea, weakness or palpitations and right heart failure may develop later in life. The defect can be closed surgically.

Patent ductus arteriosus

Patent ductus arteriosus (PDA) accounts for 10% of congenital heart defects. The ductus arteriosus connects the pulmonary artery to the descending aorta. This should close off at birth.

The PDA produces continuous shunting from the aorta to the pulmonary artery, leading to increased pulmonary venous return to the left heart and an increased left ventricular volume load. There are usually no symptoms. A continuous heart murmur is heard. An ECG and chest X-ray may show an enlarged left ventricle. Large defects lead to left ventricular failure with dyspnoea. The duct can be ligated surgically or with an umbrella occlusion device. Antibiotic prophylaxis is advised.

Pulmonary stenosis

Pulmonary stenosis accounts for about 7% of defects and may be valvular or subvalvular (infundibular). If severe there is peripheral cyanosis. Diagnosis is by the characteristic murmur, ECG and radiological changes. For severe pulmonary stenosis, balloon valvuloplasty or valvotomy is indicated.

Coarctation of the aorta

Coarctation accounts for 5–7% of congenital heart defects and is characterised by narrowing of the aorta at or just distal to the ductus arteriosus. Coarctation is a cause of secondary hypertension and is often asymptomatic. Clinically, there is a delay between the radial and the femoral pulses. When present, symptoms include headache, intermittent claudication, stroke and endocarditis. Antibiotic prophylaxis should be advised. Treatment is by surgical resection.

Summary: Congenital heart disease

- **Types**: ventricular septal defect is the most common, followed by atrial septal defect, patent ductus arteriosus, pulmonary stenosis and coarctation.
- **Treatment**: corrective surgery is usually undertaken.
- **Antibiotic prophylaxis** is required for dental treatment.

Pacemakers

Iftikhar U. Haq

Pacemakers supply an electrical stimulus to the heart to make it contract. The commonest indication for pacemaker insertion is a conduction disturbance resulting in a symptomatic bradycardia. Less commonly they are used in suppressing resistant tachyarrhythmias. The generator lies subcutaneously, most commonly under the left clavicle. From this, either one or two leads travel to the right atrium, right ventricle, or both via the subclavian vein. The pacemaker may be reprogrammed through the skin as needs change, for example the rate can be altered.

The use of ultrasonic scaling instruments and diathermy for haemostasis should be avoided during dental procedures in patients with cardiac pacemakers, as they may interfere with the pacemaker's function. If necessary, there should be continuous ECG monitoring, the diathermy should be as far away from the pacemaker as possible, and pacemaker function should be checked after the procedure.

Summary: Pacemakers

- Pacemakers **supply electrical stimulation** to the heart to make it contract, e.g. if there is a problem with the conducting system of the heart.
- **Avoid** the use of diathermy in patients with pacemakers.

Cardiomyopathy

Iftikhar U. Haq

Cardiomyopathy is a disorder of heart muscle. It is classified into three types as hypertrophic, dilated and restrictive. Hypertrophic cardiomyopathy (HCM) follows an autosomal dominant inheritance, although half occur sporadically. There is asymmetrical left ventricular hypertrophy that leads to symptoms of dyspneoa, angina, palpitations and syncope. It may be complicated by atrial fibrillation, systemic emboli, heart failure, and sudden death, the risk of which is probably increased by strenuous exercise.

In dilated (congestive) cardiomyopathy the ventricles are dilated and contract only poorly. Causes include viral and bacterial infections, alcohol, drugs, e.g. anti-cancer therapies, muscular dystrophies and infiltrations, e.g. sarcoidosis, amyloidosis and haemochromatosis. It may also be familial. Clinically, there are usually signs of right and left heart failure, cardiomegaly, and atrial fibrillation with emboli. More dangerous arrhythmias and conduction defects occur. The coronary arteries are usually normal.

Restrictive cardiomyopathy is due to endomyocardial stiffening, for which the commonest cause in the UK is amyloidosis.

Summary: Cardiomyopathy

- **Classification**: disorders of the heart muscle are divided into hypertrophic, dilated and restrictive.
- **Features**: cardiac failure and arrhythmias often occur.

Valvular heart disease

Kevin Channer

All valves in the heart are designed as one-way valves. When diseased they may either leak (incompetence) or become narrow (stenosed). Valves may be congenitally abnormal in which case they degenerate quicker than do normal valves. All valves thicken with age and may degenerate to such an extent that they require replacement.

Some diseases cause premature valve damage. They include connective tissue diseases like Marfan's syndrome or rheumatic conditions (rheumatoid arthritis or systemic lupus erythematosus). In rheumatic fever a pancarditis occurs which is associated with acute valvular incompetence. In the course of healing valves usually become scarred and then stenosed.

Pathophysiology

The pathophysiology of valve damage has important potential consequences for dentists. With stenosis or incompetence of the mitral valve, left atrial pressure increases, effectively reducing pulmonary venous return. This results in pulmonary congestion and symptoms of breathlessness and orthopnoea.

The same phenomenon occurs with aortic incompetence and stenosis but in these valve lesions the rise in intra-atrial pressure is triggered by left ventricular failure. The physical signs of valve lesions may be dramatic and are called heart murmurs.

Symptoms and consequences

Symptoms of heart failure caused by valvular heart disease makes the patient breathless and produce orthopnoea. This may limit the patient's ability to lie down, and/or make the patient uncomfortable during dental surgery. Drugs used in patients with valvular heart disease include diuretics, digoxin, and anticoagulants (e.g. warfarin) since many patients have atrial fibrillation. Strategies for dealing with dental care in anticoagulated patients need to be recognised.

Infective endocarditis

The most feared complication of valvular heart disease is endocarditis; the cutaneous signs on the nails and the fingers are shown in Colour Plate 7. When infection of the heart valves is caused by virulent organisms (e.g. *Staphylococcus*) then rapid destruction of valve tissue with severe incompetence and heart failure may ensue. This requires urgent repair and replacement of the heart valve. These infections may occur when the valve is normal. However, most infections of heart valves are subacute or chronic and are caused by organisms of low virulence (like *Streptococcus viridans*) which are common mouth commensals.

Bacterial entry into the bloodstream is increased during vigorous tooth brushing and dental treatment, especially extractions and any treatment that causes gum bleeding. Subacute infectious endocarditis only occurs in patients with pre-existing valve lesions.

Consequences for the dentist

Dental therapy may therefore expose the patient to the risk of endocarditis. As a consequence antibiotic prophylaxis prior to dental surgery is recommended. Dentists who do not follow recommendations about antibiotic prophylaxis are likely to expose themselves to a risk of litigation. Appropriate antibiotic prophylaxis strategies are listed in drug formularies such as the *British National Formulary* (see Section 3: Pharmacology and Anaesthetics).

Patients who have a prosthetic valve pose an even bigger problem because if this gets infected it must be replaced as antibiotics are usually ineffective. The antibiotic requirements for prophylaxis are stricter and may require parenteral therapy which can only usually be given in a hospital setting.

Summary: Valvular heart disease

- **Diseased heart valves** may result from congenital abnormality that leads to premature degeneration or be acquired from, for example, a connective tissue disorder or rheumatic fever.
- **Pathophysiology**: Stenosis or incompetence of the mitral valve leads to pulmonary congestion, giving rise to breathlessness. Aortic valve disease produces a rise in the intra-atrial pressure triggered by left ventricular failure.
- **Infective endocarditis** is most likely to occur on a damaged heart valve and may be caused by normal mouth commensals.

Arrhythmias

Kevin Channer

In normal individuals the heart beats in sinus rhythm (Figure 3.3). Valvular heart disease is associated with atrial fibrillation (Figure 3.4), a condition that causes a rapid and irregular heart beat which the patient feels as palpitation. Atrial fibrillation is the commonest chronic arrhythmia, occurring in about 4% of people aged over 65 years but in nearly 10% of octogenarians.

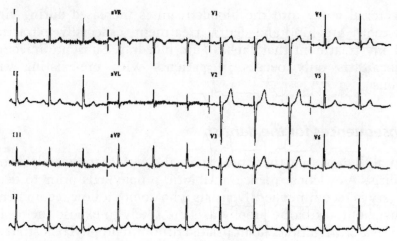

Figure 3.3 A normal electrocardiograph (ECG).

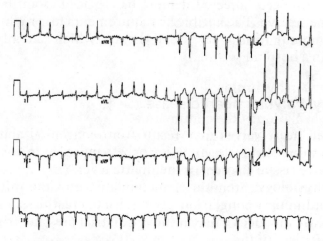

Figure 3.4 Atrial fibrillation.

The main problem with this arrhythmia is the increased risk of intracardiac clot formation and systemic embolism. For this reason patients with chronic atrial fibrillation take either aspirin or more usually warfarin as an anticoagulant. Digoxin is the most commonly used drug to reduce the tachycardia by blocking atrial conduction through the atrioventricular node.

Other cardiac arrhythmias including ectopic beats (Figure 3.5), ventricular tachycardia and bradyarrhythmias are associated with valvular and many other forms of heart disease.

Many patients experience anxiety and stress when visiting the dentist and this increases the tendency to develop tachyarrhythmias.

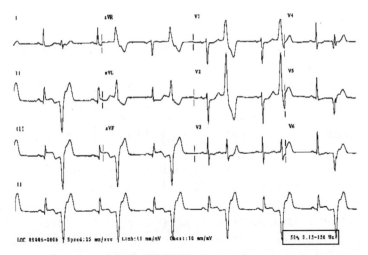

Figure 3.5 Ventricular bigeminy (paired ventricular beats).

Bradycardia may occur as part of a vasovagal reaction to stress and this may cause faintness.

Summary: Arrhythmias

- **Atrial fibrillation** is the commonest arrhythmia especially in the elderly. Affected patients are often treated with warfarin to prevent embolisation of blood clots from the heart.
- **Consequences for the dentist**: the heart patient may be on warfarin (and need their prothrombin time checking prior to dental treatment), antibiotic prophylaxis may be required if there is valvular heart disease, the patient may need to sit up during dental treatment to be comfortable if they are breathless lying down.

Hypertension

Phil S. Sanmuganathan and David J. Gawkrodger

Hypertension is very common, affecting 10–20% of the adult population. Many adults attending the dental practice will suffer from high blood pressure and be on medication for this. Many risk factors can contribute towards the development of hypertension. These include gender, age, genetic factors, alcohol, salt intake, cigarette smoking, obesity, 'stress' and the effects of some drugs such as non-steroidal analgesics, corticosteroids and the oral contraceptive pill.

Guidelines for treatment

There are now established guidelines advising physicians when and how to treat a patient with hypertension. Assessment of the patient depends not only on the blood pressure but also on other cardio-vascular risk factors such as diabetes, cigarette smoking, cholesterol level, end-organ complications and evidence of existing vascular disease. The 'normal' blood pressure is 120/80 mm Hg (systolic over diastolic).

Treatment of blood pressure is recommended when there is a systolic of 160–199 or diastolic of 100–109, sustained over 4–12 weeks, without evidence of target organ damage, diabetes or cardiovascular complications. Treatment is suggested at lower levels if hypertension persists and the patient's risk for coronary heart disease has been assessed at 15% over the next 10 years. The optimal target systolic pressure is ≤140, and diastolic ≤85.

Organ damage

Early and effective treatment is aimed at reducing the risk of the complications of having a high blood pressure. Hypertension can have a serious effect on the cerebrovascular circulation, with the development of thrombotic and haemorrhagic strokes, hypertensive encephalopathy and even dementia. The cardiac effects of a high blood pressure are left ventricular hypertrophy, coronary artery disease and cardiac failure. Prolonged hypertension may result in kidney damage, impaired renal function and retinopathy.

Benefits of intervention

Most patients with hypertension are asymptomatic. In 5% there is a secondary cause and investigation is required to detect this. In 'malignant' hypertension, without treatment, there is a mortality of 100% within two years: this falls to less than 5% when the raised blood pressure is treated. For moderate hypertension, a 48% reduction in strokes and a 16% fall in coronary heart disease have been shown with treatment.

Therapy

A thiazide diuretic is usually the first line treatment. Beta blockers, calcium channel blockers, and ACE inhibitors are often prescribed. Non-pharmacological measures such as weight reduction, reduced dietary intake of salt and alcohol, exercise and cessation of smoking are often recommended. Other drugs used include alpha adrenergic blocking drugs, vasodilators, angiotensin II receptor antagonists and centrally acting antihypertensives.

Summary: Hypertension

• **Risk factors** for hypertension include family history of hypertension, obesity, excess alcohol, smoking, stress and the effects of some drugs, e.g. steroids.
• **Guidelines** are available: a sustained systolic BP of 160–199 or a diastolic BP of 100–109 in a patient with no complicating factors should be treated.
• **Target blood pressure** is systolic ≤140, diastolic ≤85.
• **Target organ damage** includes stroke, cardiac failure, coronary artery disease, renal impairment and retinopathy.
• **Symptoms**: most patients are asymptomatic, hypertension is common affecting 10–20% of adults, detected by measuring blood pressure.
• **Intervention** is to reduce mortality and morbidity from cardiovascular complications.
• **Treatment** is initially with a thiazide diuretic, often with a beta blocker, ACE inhibitor, calcium-channel blocker added.

Further reading

British Hypertension Society (1999) Guidelines for the management of hypertension: report of the third working party of the British Hypertension Society. *J Hum Hypertens* 13: 569–92.
Gibbs, C.R., Davies, M.K., Lip, G.V.H. (2000) *ABC of Heart Failure*. London, BMJ Books.
Hough, R., Haq, I.U. (1999) Congenital heart disease. In (Hough, R., & Haq, I.U. eds.) *Internal Medicine*. London, Mosby, 222–4.

Websites

Ischaemic heart disease:
    http://www.wikipedia.org/wiki/ischaemic_heart_disease
Congenital heart disease: http://www.csun.edu/~hcmth011/heart/
American Society of Hypertension: http://www.ash-us.org

CHAPTER 4
Respiratory Diseases

Respiratory symptoms are common and dentists need to know when a patient is in respiratory distress and what to do when this occurs.

Chronic obstructive airways disease

Rod Lawson

Chronic obstructive airways disease (COAD) or chronic bronchitis is a clinical diagnosis. It is the production of sputum on most days for three months per year, on two successive years. Emphysema is the destruction of the alveolar walls (Figure 4.1). Chronic bronchitis and emphysema often co-exist. The generic term 'chronic obstructive pulmonary disease' (COPD, sometimes also called chronic obstructive airways disease or chronic obstructive lung disease) is often used. COPD gives rise to airflow obstruction, as quantified by the forced expiratory volume in one second (FEV1).

Dyspnoea is the sensation of breathlessness. Cyanosis is a blue appearance of the tongue secondary to poor arterial oxygenation. The predominant cause of COPD is smoking. Alpha 1-antitrypsin deficiency is an inherited disorder that makes individuals more likely to get emphysema.

Clinical features

The cardinal feature of COPD is dyspnoea secondary to airflow obstruction (Table 4.1). This occurs on exertion and is relieved by rest, except that in late stage disease, dyspnoea at rest may be present. Symptoms vary little from day to day but exacerbations may occur, with progressive increase in breathlessness for a period

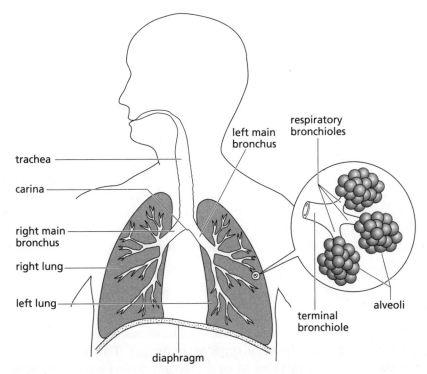

Figure 4.1 The structure of the respiratory tract.

Table 4.1 Clinical features of common respiratory diseases

Condition	Symptoms
asthma	wheeze cough dyspnoea diurnal variation (worst in morning) nocturnal awakening with dyspnoea postexertional wheeze symptoms vary day-to-day
chronic obstructive airways disease	dyspnoea with wheeze cough +/– sputum steady deterioration of symptoms with little variation weight loss can be a feature
lung cancer	haemoptysis with chronic cough new/unexplained dyspnoea malaise anorexia weight loss local chest pain hoarse voice (recurrent laryngeal nerve palsy) symptoms of metastases in bone, brain, liver, adrenals

of days. Cough with or without sputum may be present. The sputum is usually pale. Yellow or green suggests infection, blood raises the possibility of lung cancer. As smoking causes both lung cancer and COPD, the two often co-exist. In advanced COPD there may be weight loss and weakness. Patients may be breathless and tend to have a large, hyperexpanded chest (see Colour Plate 9), with an increased respiratory rate. Wheezes may be audible.

The degree of a patient's functional ability should be assessed by questions about everyday life, e.g. how far they can walk, whether they can climb a flight of stairs without stopping, whether they can go out and do their shopping. Formal measurement of lung function allows an objective measure of severity. It is important to be aware of the possibility of co-existent cardiac disease (suggested by chest pain on exertion, breathlessness on lying flat and ankle swelling).

Treatment

Inhalers delivering beta 2 agonists (e.g. salbutamol) or anticholinergics (e.g. ipratropium) are the mainstays of treatment. Theophyllines (e.g. aminophylline) and inhaled or oral steroids may be used. Severely affected patients may require long-term oxygen therapy.

Specific dental considerations

Breathless patients often experience difficulty brushing their teeth. They should do this seated and after rest, and may need to brush one portion of the teeth at a time. Inhaled steroids may be associated with oral candida. Use of spacer devices with inhalers and gargling with water after taking steroid inhalers reduce the incidence of this. Weight loss may lead to poorly fitting dentures, further reducing oral intake, and exacerbating the problem. Mouth breathing may dry the mouth giving problems with oral hygiene. COPD patients who smoke are at risk of oral cancers.

Dental treatment of a patient with COPD should be deferred during an exacerbation unless there is an emergency. If there is doubt as to the patient's stability, or as to the presence of co-morbidities, the patient should be referred to their general medical practitioner for further advice. Patients should take their usual reliever inhaler 20–30 minutes before treatment to relieve dyspnoea during the procedure.

Dyspnoeic patients will be more comfortable treated upright in the dental chair. Although patients on long-term oxygen should continue to receive supplemental oxygen during treatment, it is essential that oxygen therapy is cautious. In these patients, oxygen should be given by nasal cannulae at 1 or 2 l/min or low concentration masks (24 or 28%).

Normally, increased arterial carbon dioxide leads to increased ventilation. This mechanism may be lost in COPD, with hypoxia providing the stimulus to breathe. Administration of oxygen may abolish this stimulus with disastrous consequences. The altered respiratory drive also makes the administration of sedatives hazardous, and recovery after general anaesthesia may be poor. Sedation should only be used after specialist advice, and general anaesthesia avoided in more severely affected patients unless essential.

Summary: Chronic obstructive airways disease

• **Symptoms**: Chronic obstructive airways disease is characterised by dyspnoea with or without cough and sputum.
• **Associated cancers**: There is an increased co-existence of carcinomas of the head, neck and bronchus.
• **Management**: Treatment is with inhaled bronchodilators (with or without inhaled or oral steroids) and long-term oxygen therapy.
• **Bronchodilators**: Patients should receive inhaled bronchodilators before treatment and can be given oxygen at the rate they receive at home.
• **Avoid**: Sedation and general anaesthesia are avoided.

Pulmonary fibrosis including sarcoidosis

Rod Lawson

Cryptogenic pulmonary fibrosis (called CFA in the UK, idiopathic pulmonary fibrosis in the USA) is the name given to an autoimmune inflammatory disease of unknown cause leading to diffuse pulmonary fibrosis (scarring of the lungs). Similar conditions occur in autoimmune diseases such as rheumatoid arthritis. Sarcoidosis is a granulomatous disorder that may give rise to pulmonary fibrosis. It may affect any organ but frequently involves intrathoracic lymph nodes.

Extrinsic allergic alveolitis (EAA) is a fibrotic lung disease resulting from a specific allergy to an inhaled substance. The cause of CFA is unknown, though genetic and environmental risk factors have been identified. The cause of sarcoidosis is also uncertain but the allergen provoking EAA can usually be identified. In asbestosis there is fibrosis of the lungs as a consequence of the inhalation of asbestos fibres. Carcinoma of the lung and mesothelioma of the pleura may result.

Clinical features

Patients will be breathless on exercise. At later stages they will be breathless at rest. They may have a dry cough or cyanosis and often have clubbing. There may be features of associated disease such as rheumatoid arthritis. Sarcoidosis may give swollen lymph nodes and salivary glands. CFA gives crackles in the chest; sarcoidosis usually does not. The degree of a patient's functional ability should be assessed by questions about everyday life. Formal spirometry will quantify the patient's disease.

Treatment

If pulmonary fibrosis is active and progressive, steroids will often be given, initially at high doses. Other immunosuppressant therapy (e.g. cyclophosphamide or azathioprine) may also be used. End-stage patients receive oxygen.

Specific dental considerations

Dyspnoeic patients may have difficulty brushing their teeth. They should rest before brushing, and remain seated, brushing the teeth in stages if necessary. CFA may be associated with the sicca syndrome, producing a pathologically dry mouth. Artificial saliva may be required. The use of steroids and immunosuppressive agents increases the risks of infection as a cause of dental problems, and as a result of surgical treatment. Immunosuppressives may cause blood dyscrasias, which may present as oral ulceration or bleeding. Dyspnoeic patients will be more comfortable treated sitting.

Summary: Pulmonary fibrosis including sarcoidosis

• **Cryptogenic fibrosing alveolitis** is characterised by breathlessness, clubbing and crackles, and may be treated with steroids and oxygen. Steroid cover may be needed for some procedures.
• In **sarcoidosis** people experience breathlessness without clubbing or crackles.
• **Treatment**: Pulmonary fibrosis may be treated with steroids and oxygen, and steroid cover may be needed for certain procedures.

Cystic fibrosis

Cystic fibrosis is an inherited recessive condition in which bronchial and pancreatic secretions are abnormally viscous. The sweat has a high sodium content. It presents in childhood with repeated respiratory infections that result from the blockage of the bronchial tree by viscous mucus. Infective complications ensue.

Patients often have associated pancreatic disease and may be poorly nourished. They may show swelling of salivary glands. Treatment is aimed at general support, controlling respiratory infection, maintaining lung function and prescribing pancreatin (pancreatic enzymes) to assist digestion. Lung transplant is a treatment.

If the patient is in respiratory failure, the dentist should enquire if they are more comfortable sitting up. They might require oxygen or the use of bronchodilators. If the patient has had a lung transplant they will be on immunosuppressive drugs, which predispose to infection or possibly bleeding.

Carcinoma of the bronchus

Bronchial carcinoma is one of the commonest cancers. It is more common in men but the incidence in women is rising. Cigarette smoking is a well-recognised cause but other associations include exposure to asbestos, and some atmospheric pollutants.

Clinical features

Cough or worsening of an existing cough is often a presenting symptom. Other manifestations include coughing up blood (haemoptysis), shortness of breath, central chest ache, pleuritic chest pain or slow resolution of a chest infection. Metastases may involve the liver, brain, skin or adrenal glands.

Local extension of the tumour can result in obstruction of the superior vena cava (giving plethoric and persisting swelling of the face and neck), hoarseness due to palsy of the recurrent laryngeal nerve, or enlarged lymph nodes in the neck. The chest X-ray often shows a mass. Examination of the bronchial tree using a bronchoscope (with biopsy) confirms the diagnosis.

Treatment

Excision of the cancer is the desired management if it is resectable. Other approaches include radiotherapy and chemotherapy. There are unlikely to be specific considerations for the dentist, although attention should be paid to whether the patient is malnourished, or receiving chemotherapy or radiotherapy, which might make them more prone to infection or bleeding.

Summary: Cystic fibrosis and carcinoma of the bronchus

• **Cystic fibrosis** is a recessively inherited condition that affects mucus secreting glands: it results in respiratory infections, pancreatic disease and malnourishment. Respiratory failure is the end result. If there has been a lung transplant, consideration of the effects of immunosuppressive drugs is needed.

• **Carcinoma of the bronchus** is a common cancer. Patients receiving dental treatment may be at risk of infection or bleeding if they are receiving chemotherapy or radiotherapy.

Asthma

Paul B. Anderson

Asthma is defined on the basis of variable airflow obstruction, either spontaneously with time, or in response to treatment.

Clinical features

Airway inflammation leads to hyper-reactivity, wheezing, dyspnoea, sputum production and cough. Asthma may start at any age and affects 10% of the population. Early onset tends to be allergic (e.g. house dust mite, animals, pollen) and to be associated with hay fever and eczema (atopy).

Later onset asthma is less often associated with allergy but may be precipitated by physical stimuli such as exercise, cold air, fumes, dust, irritants and viruses. These physical stimuli will also cause bronchoconstriction and exacerbation of symptoms in allergic asthmatics. Some drugs, e.g. aspirin and nonsteroidal anti-inflammatories, can precipitate bronchoconstriction.

Treatment

The treatment of asthma is usually with a combination of broncho-dilator (reliever) and anti-inflammatory (preventer) drugs. These are given by inhalation rather than orally. Direct delivery to the respiratory tract leads to a more rapid response, greater effectiveness and fewer side effects. There are a variety of inhalation devices (metered dose inhalers, dry powder inhalers, and nebulisers). The patient must understand how to use the device correctly (Figure 4.2). The bronchodilators include the beta agonists (e.g. salbutamol), the anticholinergics (e.g. ipratropium), and the xanthines (e.g.

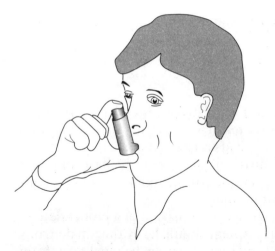

Remove the dust cap, shake the inhaler, hold the inhaler upright with your thumb on the base. Breathe out steadily as far as is comfortable but not completely. Place the mouthpiece in your mouth and close your lips around it.
Start to breathe in through your mouth and press down on the top of the inhaler.
Continue to breathe in steadily and deeply.
Hold your breath for as long as comfortable, about ten seconds.

Figure 4.2 How to use an inhaler.

aminophylline). The anti-inflammatory or prophylactic drugs include the cromones (e.g. sodium cromoglycate), the inhaled steroids (e.g. beclomethasone) and the leucotriene receptor antagonists (e.g. montelukast).

When asthma is mild and intermittent, an occasional dose of bronchodilator may be all that is required. However, most asthmatics require regular anti-inflammatory treatment, usually an inhaled steroid, and as required bronchodilator. Education, avoidance of precipitating factors, and efforts to ensure compliance are also helpful. An acute asthma is treated with high dose bronchodilators given by inhaler and spacer or nebuliser, steroids (hydrocortisone or prednisolone), oxygen and antibiotics if there is evidence of respiratory infection. Hospital admission is often required. Severe acute asthma may require ventilation.

Specific dental considerations

Oxygen should be available at each dental practice with a selection of masks and nasal cannulae. It would be advantageous to have some bronchodilator inhalers and large volume spacers to use in patients with asthma or COPD but many of these patients will be carrying their own inhalers. A nebuliser and bronchodilator solution would be useful for those who find it difficult to use a spacer when distressed.

Oxygen is used to correct hypoxia and improve tissue oxygenation. In most cases of acute breathlessness, for example in asthma and heart failure, oxygen should be given at high concentrations by mask (60–100%). In hospital, hypoxia is detected and treatment monitored by pulse oximetry and by measuring arterial blood gases.

Summary: Asthma

- **Symptoms**: Dyspnoea can result from respiratory or cardiac causes, but wheezing suggests a respiratory origin. A chest X-ray can differentiate many non-wheezy causes from cardiac ones.
- **Asthma** is a common condition diagnosed on the basis of reversible airflow obstruction. It is eminently treatable but nevertheless many asthmatics remain symptomatic.
- **Management**: Therapy is with a combination of a bronchodilator and an anti-inflammatory. Treatment should be by the inhaled route but devices must be selected and their use must be taught carefully.

Pulmonary embolism

Paul B. Anderson

Thrombus may form in the deep veins in the legs (deep vein thrombosis, DVT) or the pelvis and embolise to the lungs where it may obstruct the pulmonary arterial circulation and may result in pulmonary infarction. Classic symptoms are dyspnoea, pleuritic chest pain and haemoptysis – but significant emboli can occur in the absence of pain or haemoptysis. If the pulmonary circulation is severely compromised the patient may become shocked.

In most patients there is a predisposing factor, such as trauma, surgery, immobility, malignancy, obesity, age, pregnancy/puerperium, disabling disease, previous pulmonary embolism or DVT or thrombotic tendency including oral contraceptive use. The diagnosis requires clinical suspicion and appropriate tests, e.g. a lung perfusion scan or a spiral computed tomography (CT) scan. Treatment is with oxygen, circulatory support, analgesics and anticoagulation, initially with heparin, then with warfarin. In severe cases thrombolytic drugs are indicated.

Summary: Pulmonary emboli

- **Pulmonary emboli** are an important cause of morbidity and mortality and may be difficult to diagnose but attention to prophylactic measures in high risk groups can substantially reduce the risk of fatal events.
- **Oxygen** is indicated in acute dyspnoea but care must be taken in COPD.

Chest pain of respiratory origin

Steve R. Brennan

A patient may develop chest pain during dental treatment and so a dentist needs to have a good idea of how to cope with the situation when it occurs. Chest pains may be of cardiac, respiratory, musculo-skeletal or gastrointestinal origin.

It can be difficult to make a definitive diagnosis in an acute situation in a dental practice. Specific points to note on examination include:

- is the patient distressed?
- are they pale and sweaty? (might suggest a cardiac cause)
- is the pulse rapid? (may indicate a cardiac or cardiopulmonary origin)
- are they breathless? (suggests either cardiac or pulmonary cause)
- is there a tender area on the chest wall? (might indicate a rib fracture or musculoskeletal cause).

Often the findings may suggest more than one possible diagnosis. In pleurisy, due to irritation of the pleura of the lungs in pneumonia, there is usually quite good localisation by the patient to a particular part of the chest wall and the pain is worse with coughing. However, a 'cracked' rib may give an identical presentation.

Small pulmonary emboli can give rise to pleurisy, a medium-sized pulmonary embolus can result in breathlessness without chest pain, but larger pulmonary emboli produce cardiac-type pain with collapse and possible death. In bronchitis or tracheitis, there is soreness in the centre of the chest, behind the sternum, and the symptoms are worse with coughing. Nonetheless, angina or myocardial infarction need to be considered.

Pneumothorax may also be a cause of chest pain. Oesophageal pain from reflux oesophagitis can be confusing as the pain may be retrosternal, and worse on bending or lying down.

Summary: Chest pain of respiratory origin

- **Diagnosis**: The differential diagnosis of chest pain includes cardiac, pulmonary, gastrointestinal and musculoskeletal causes. Differentiating between them is often not easy.
- **Differentiation by history**: History is useful and may indicate respiratory origin, e.g. pleuritic pain, cardiac cause, e.g. pain radiates down the arm, or gastrointestinal, e.g. retrosternal and worse on bending down.
- **Physical findings**: **Examination**, even if basic, may be revealing: circulatory collapse would suggest a cardiac cause and a tender area over a rib might indicate a fractured rib.

Further reading

Bourke, S.J., Brewis, R.A.L. (1998) *Lecture Notes on Respiratory Medicine*. 5th edition. Oxford, Blackwell Science.

Websites

Asthma: http://www.embbs.com/cr/asthma/asthmarh.html
Chest pain: http://www.madsci.com/manu/indxches.htm
Chronic obstructive airways disease:
   http://bmj.com/cgi/collection/chronic_obstructive_airways

CHAPTER 5
Gastrointestinal Diseases

The oral cavity is the uppermost extension of the gut (Figure 5.1). Several diseases of the gastrointestinal tract have oral manifestations and so it is important for dentists to be familiar with these conditions. The major symptoms and causes are given here together with some important diseases. Other relevant conditions are shown in Table 5.1.

Symptoms of gastrointestinal disorders

Dysphagia

Swallowing is co-ordinated by the brain stem via nerves supplying the mouth, pharynx and oesophagus. Dysphagia (difficulty in swallowing) can arise from problems in any of the three phases of swallowing. The oral phase involves propelling the bolus of food into the pharynx using the tongue against the hard palate. Dental or salivary gland disorders will interfere with the preparation of food of the appropriate consistency.

Candidiasis, herpes simplex or tumours may cause painful mastication. Neurological disorders such as Parkinson's disease and motor neuron disease can affect the muscles of mastication and tongue movement and impair the initiation of swallowing.

During the pharyngeal phase of swallowing, the respiratory pathway is closed by elevation of the larynx and retroversion of the epiglottis over the laryngeal orifice. The nasopharynx is occluded by elevation of the soft palate. The bolus is propelled into the oesophagus by sequential contractions of the tongue and pharynx. The upper oesophageal sphincter relaxes transiently to allow the bolus through. As in the oral phase, local infections or tumours may impair this process.

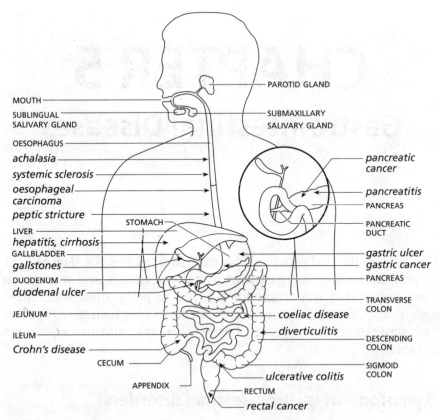

Figure 5.1 The digestive tract showing the sites of involvement of certain gastrointestinal disorders.

A pharyngeal pouch, which is a diverticulum through a dehiscence at the back of the pharynx, may give rise to regurgitation or obstruction. Coughing, choking and nasal regurgitation suggest a brain stem disorder affecting laryngeal or nasopharyngeal closure, and include cerebrovascular disease and motor neuron disease.

The oesophageal phase consists of a peristaltic wave that propels the bolus through the lower oesophageal sphincter into the stomach. Muscle or nerve disorders interfering with this co-ordinated contraction may cause dysphagia. A mechanical obstruction can be benign or malignant. In Plummer–Vinson syndrome a postcricoid web is associated with glossitis, angular cheilitis, koilonychia (see Colour Plate 3) and iron deficiency. Older individuals with oesophageal diverticulae or pharyngeal pouches may present with dysphagia, regurgitation, pulmonary aspiration or a palpable neck swelling after eating. Recent onset of dysphagia and weight loss in an elderly person should, however, signify carcinoma until proven otherwise.

Table 5.1 Clinical features of gastrointestinal disorders

Disease	Mechanism or cause where known	Clinical features
Oesophageal disease		
webs/rings	congenital, iron deficiency	dysphagia
diverticulae/pouches	motility disorder, previous inflammation in oesophagus or mediastinum	regurgitation, pulmonary aspiration
achalasia	failure of lower oesophageal sphincter to relax	dysphagia, regurgitation, weight loss
systemic sclerosis	oesophageal peristaltic failure and low lower oesophageal sphincter pressure	dysphagia, heartburn
gastro-oesophageal reflux disease (GORD)	excessive and prolonged relaxation of lower oesophageal sphincter	heartburn and acid reflux
benign peptic (reflux) stricture	prolonged exposure to gastric acid and pepsin due to GORD	dysphagia
oesophageal carcinoma		dysphagia and weight loss
Gastroduodenal disease		
functional dyspepsia	abnormalities in gastric nerve and muscle function, acid sensitivity	epigastric pain, distension, nausea
gastric ulcer	non-steroidal anti-inflammatory drugs, *H. pylori*	epigastric pain, vomiting, weight loss
duodenal ulcer	*H. pylori*	epigastric pain
gastric carcinoma	*H. pylori*	epigastric pain, vomiting, weight loss
Small intestinal disease		
coeliac disease	gluten sensitivity	anaemia, asymptomatic or diarrhoea, weight loss
Crohn's disease		diarrhoea, pain, weight loss

Table 5.1 *(cont'd)*

Disease	Mechanism or cause where known	Clinical features
Hepatobiliary disease		
gallstones		severe episodic right upper quadrant/epigastric pain; fever and jaundice if stone in bile duct
viral hepatitis	hepatitis A, B	anorexia, malaise, fever, jaundice
cirrhosis	alcohol, chronic viral hepatitis B or C, genetic haemochromatosis, autoimmune hepatitis, primary biliary cirrhosis	upper gastrointestinal bleeding, abdominal distension (ascites), leg swelling (oedema), jaundice
Pancreatic disease		
pancreatitis	alcohol, gallstones, hypercalcaemia, hyperlipidaemia, familial	episodic severe upper abdominal pain, vomiting, fever, jaundice
pancreatic carcinoma		constant upper abdominal pain, weight loss, jaundice
Colorectal disease		
ulcerative colitis		diarrhoea with blood and mucus per rectum
Crohn's disease		diarrhoea, abdominal pain, weight loss
diverticulitis	inflammation in diverticulae	left iliac fossa pain, fever, tenderness
colorectal cancer		change in bowel habit (diarrhoea and/or constipation), abdominal pain, weight loss, rectal bleeding
Other		
irritable bowel syndrome	motility disorder affecting gastrointestinal tract	abdominal pain, diarrhoea and/or constipation, mucus per rectum, bloating; often longstanding symptoms

Investigation is by radiological contrast (barium) studies and endoscopy. Endoscopic bougie dilation is effective treatment for webs and rings but surgery is the treatment of choice for pouches and early cancers.

Upper abdominal pain

Dyspepsia is defined as pain or discomfort centred in the upper abdomen. Nausea, vomiting, anorexia and distension are commonly associated symptoms. The majority of patients (60%) have functional (or non-ulcer) dyspepsia, in which no easily definable cause is found. Of the rest, approximately 20% have a peptic (duodenal or gastric) ulcer, 15% have gastro-oesophageal reflux and about 1–2% have gastric or pancreatic cancer.

Disorders of the hepatobiliary system and pancreas may present with similar symptoms. Benign disorders (gallstones and pancreatitis: see Table 5.1) tend to cause episodic severe pain, and pancreatic cancer causes an unremitting pain often with weight loss and jaundice.

Investigation is by upper gastrointestinal endoscopy and/or ultrasound and computed tomography (CT) scanning. If ulcers are suspected, tests for *Helicobacter pylori* infection may be performed as all duodenal ulcers are associated with infection as well as gastric ulcers in which non-steroidal anti-inflammatory drugs are not implicated. Peptic ulcers are treated with acid suppressant drugs and antibiotics to eradicate *H. pylori* infection where appropriate. Gastro-oesophageal reflux is managed using antacids or acid suppressants. Surgery is indicated for most gallstones or gastrointestinal cancer.

Jaundice

Bilirubin is derived from haem released by breakdown of damaged red blood cells. It is metabolised and excreted by the liver via the bile ducts into the duodenum. When present in excess, bilirubin may be deposited in the skin and ocular sclerae, giving rise to jaundice.

Pre-hepatic jaundice may be due to the rapid destruction of abnormal red cells (haemolytic anaemia). Hepatic jaundice is due to liver disease and might be caused by infections (e.g. hepatitis A), drugs (particularly antibiotics), alcohol or one of the chronic liver diseases (cirrhosis). Post-hepatic jaundice is usually due to obstruction of the bile duct by gallstones (often associated with severe abdominal pain and fever) or cancer of the pancreas or bile duct.

Jaundice requires urgent medical attention, so dental treatment should be postponed or undertaken only in close co-operation with the patient's medical specialist. Most patients with chronic liver disease or cirrhosis, however, are not jaundiced. The commonest cause is alcohol, but there are several other common causes of cirrhosis (Table 5.1).

Of immediate relevance to dental practice is that the liver is responsible for the manufacture of clotting proteins, so patients with cirrhosis may have bleeding tendencies. Those most at risk are patients who have advanced or decompensated liver disease, signs of which include jaundice, weight loss, ascites (fluid accumulation in the abdomen), peripheral oedema (swollen legs), mental dullness or confusion or recent gastrointestinal bleeding. The coagulation status can be readily assessed by measuring the prothrombin and partial thromboplastin times. These may be prolonged in liver disease due to deficiency of vitamin K (which is necessary for the synthesis of several clotting factors). Bleeding tendencies may be exacerbated by a low platelet count, a common feature of cirrhosis.

Patients should be advised to abstain from alcohol before procedures and the administration of vitamin K may improve the prothrombin time. Failure to correct clotting abnormalities with vitamin K might require treatment with infusions of clotting factors.

Jaundice is investigated initially using blood tests and radiological imaging of the liver and bile ducts. Blood tests may reveal evidence of infection or specific liver diseases (see Table 5.1). The bile ducts are dilated on ultrasound scanning if obstruction is the cause. Viral hepatitis usually resolves spontaneously. Drug-related or alcoholic hepatitis usually improves when exposure to the injurious agent ceases. Biliary obstruction should be relieved either endoscopically or surgically.

Gastrointestinal diseases of importance to dentists

Inflammatory bowel disease

Ulcerative colitis and Crohn's disease are the chronic idiopathic inflammatory bowel diseases which commonly present in young people. Ulcerative colitis affects the rectum and part or all of the colon. Diarrhoea with blood and mucus per rectum is a common symptom. Crohn's disease most frequently affects the terminal ileum and caecum, but can affect any part of the gastrointestinal tract from lips to anus. Symptoms include diarrhoea, abdominal pain and weight loss.

Oral aphthous ulceration is frequently associated with active inflammatory bowel disease. Crohn's disease occasionally causes deep ulcers, fissuring and cobblestoning in the oral mucosa or diffuse swelling of the lips and cheek (see Colour Plates 14 and 15).

Investigation is by colonoscopy and barium contrast studies of the small and large bowel. Steroids are used to treat active disease and several anti-inflammatory and immunosuppressive agents are used to maintain remission. Surgery is an important treatment option for many.

Coeliac disease

Coeliac disease affects about 1 in 300 of the population and commonly presents in the younger age groups. A reaction to the protein gluten (in wheat, barley and rye) causes injury to the small intestinal mucosa which may result in diarrhoea and weight loss. However, many patients have few symptoms and present only when malabsorption of iron and folic acid has caused anaemia. Oral aphthous ulcers also occur in coeliac disease. Serum antibody tests (antigliadin and antiendomysial) are widely used to screen for coeliac disease, but definitive diagnosis is made by histological examination of endoscopic duodenal biopsies. Symptoms resolve on a gluten-free diet.

Gastrointestinal cancer

The rectum and the colon are the commonest sites for gastrointestinal cancer, affecting 1 in 100 people usually in the over 60 age group. A change in bowel habit (diarrhoea and/or constipation), abdominal pain, rectal bleeding and weight loss are common symptoms. Other gastrointestinal cancers are discussed above. Suspected colorectal cancer needs urgent investigation by colonoscopy or barium contrast studies. Surgery is the mainstay of treatment.

Summary: Gastrointestinal diseases

- **Dysphagia** may be due to inflammatory, neurological or malignant disease affecting the oral, pharyngeal or oesophageal phase of swallowing.
- **Dyspepsia** is common and usually benign. Peptic ulcer, gastro-oesophageal reflux and gallstones can be easily treated.
- **Jaundice** requires urgent investigation to determine the cause. It may be associated with clotting abnormalities.
- **Inflammatory bowel disease** typically causes diarrhoea, abdominal pain, weight loss and rectal bleeding in young adults. Oral aphthous ulcers occur in ulcerative colitis, but Crohn's disease may specifically affect the buccal mucosa, lips and cheeks.
- **Coeliac disease** classically presents as diarrhoea, weight loss and anaemia but many patients are relatively asymptomatic. Oral aphthous ulcers may occur.

• **Gastrointestinal cancer** should be suspected in any older patient with gastrointestinal symptoms and weight loss.

Further reading

Misiewicz, J.J., Pounder, R.E., Venables, C.W. (eds) (1994) *Diseases of the Gut and Pancreas*. 2nd edition. Oxford, Blackwell Science.

Sherlock, S., Dooley, J. (1996) *Diseases of the Liver and Biliary System*, 10th edition, Oxford, Blackwell Science.

Websites

Gut Online: http://gut.bmjjournals.com
Gastrohep: http://www.gastrohep.com
Gastroenterology: http://intl.gastrojournal.org

CHAPTER 6
Endocrinological Diseases and Diabetes

Endocrine diseases are common and many dental patients are on hormone replacement. In this section, thyroid, adrenal and pituitary disease will be outlined, and diabetes will be discussed.

Thyroid disease

The thyroid gland is situated anterior to the thyroid cartilage in the neck. The thyroid gland synthesises, stores and releases thyroid hormone in the forms T_3 and T_4. The formation of these hormones is intricately dependent on the trapping of iodine by the thyroid gland and its subsequent organification into the hormone. T_4 is produced entirely by the thyroid while T_3 is mainly produced by peripheral conversion from T_4 in cells of the kidney, liver, heart, anterior pituitary, and other tissues. It is the T_3 hormone that is mainly biologically active.

These hormones pass through the circulation bound to serum proteins including thyroxine-binding globulin and albumin. It is the level of free hormones that govern the metabolic state and thyroid status of a patient.

Biochemistry

The synthesis and release of thyroxine is under the influence of thyroid stimulating hormone (TSH) which is released from the anterior pituitary, and this in turn is released under the influence of thyrotrophic releasing hormone (TRH) which is secreted by the hypothalamus (Figure 6.1). Thyroxine feeds back to switch off the release of TRH and TSH in a classic endocrine feedback loop.

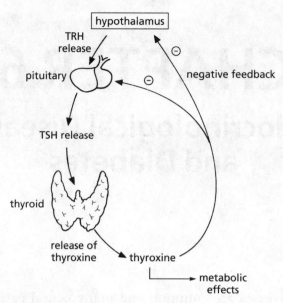

Figure 6.1 The hypothalamic-thyroid axis.

Elevated levels of thyroid hormone result in a suppression of TSH. This fact forms the mainstay of the biochemical assessment of the thyroid status. As the signs and symptoms of thyroid dysfunction can be extremely non-specific, the clinical decisions are usually based upon the reliance of a good laboratory assay for TSH, free T_3 and free T_4.

Thyroid function tests

In primary hypothyroidism, where a thyroid gland has ceased to work, untreated patients will have low circulating levels of free T_4 and free T_3. Consequently there will be no feedback at the pituitary and hypothalamic levels and the level of TSH will rise. In contrast, in primary overactivity of the thyroid gland, leading to hyper-thyroidism, high levels of circulating thyroid hormone will suppress the circulating levels of TSH. This demonstrates the central role of TSH estimation and determining whether a patient has either an underactive or overactive thyroid gland. A normal TSH effectively excludes primary hypo- or hyperthyroidism.

Primary hypothyroidism

By far the commonest cause of primary hypothyroidism is thyroid destruction by autoimmunity. Patients commonly have a positive family history and are frequently diagnosed following symptoms of tiredness, weight gain, constipation, dryness of skin and hair, cold intolerance, hoarseness of voice, abnormal menses (frequently with menorrhagia), see Colour Plate 20. Once diagnosed with an elevated TSH and low circulating thyroxine, patients placed on thyroxine therapy are usually stable at a set dose for life. Even when mildly hypothyroid and not fully treated, patients tolerate surgical intervention well.

Hyperthyroidism

The common causes of hyperthyroidism in the adult include Graves' disease, toxic nodular goitre and toxic adenoma. Of these by far the most common is Graves' disease, which is associated with the physical signs of exophthalmos (see Colour Plate 21). Any cause of hyperthyroidism will cause lid retraction because of spasm of the levator palpabrae superioris as a result of sympathetic hyperactivity.

Symptoms of hyperthyroidism include weight loss, lack of energy, heat intolerance, anxiety and irritability, increased sweating, an increased appetite and palpitations. There may also be diarrhoea. Signs include goitre, tremor, moist hands and skin with tachycardia and restlessness. Signs specific to Graves' disease include proptosis and other eye signs (but not lid lag), thyroid acropachy and pretibial myxoedema.

Biochemically, the TSH will be suppressed with either an elevated free T_4 and/or free T_3. It is important to recognise that the eye signs of Graves' disease do not change in parallel with thyroid function. For dental practice the importance of recognising hyperthyroidism is not only to alert the GP or endocrinologist to its presence so that it may be treated adequately, but also to avoid any general anaesthetic. A patient with hyperthyroidism subjected to general anaesthesia may well suffer a thyroid storm, which is associated with a high level of mortality.

Calcium homeostasis

Serum calcium is maintained within a narrow physiological range. Calcium is bound to circulating proteins, predominantly albumin. The measurement of serum calcium has to take account of this and the value corrected for the serum albumin, with most labs reporting a corrected calcium of 2.2–2.6 mmol/l. The daily flux of calcium is intricately dependent on the actions of vitamin D and parathormone (PTH). The skeleton provides a large reservoir of calcium. Dietary vitamin D, or that formed in the skin, is hydroxylated in the liver and then the kidney to form active 1,25 dihydroxyvitamin D. This is important for the absorption of calcium from the gut and calcification of bone.

The hydroxylation of vitamin D and reabsorption of bone is stimulated by PTH. Minute to minute control of serum calcium concentration is probably achieved by fine regulation of renal calcium handling, itself dependent on 1,25 dihydroxyvitamin D, PTH and renal sodium status. Under normal circumstances the parathyroid will sense a low serum calcium and stimulate PTH secretion, while a high serum calcium will suppress PTH secretion.

Hypocalcaemia and vitamin D deficiency

Deficiency of vitamin D in childhood leads to rickets, and the weak bones give rise to the classic 'bowed leg appearance'. In adults deficiency leads to osteomalacia with bone pain and an elevated serum alkaline phosphatase. In severe deficiency hypocalcaemia may result with symptoms of weakness, tetany and carpopedal spasm. Deficiency of PTH, most commonly following neck surgery for thyroid disease, results in hypocalcaemia. Severe hypocalcaemia, serum calcium <1.8 mmol/l, can be life threatening and requires urgent investigation and treatment.

Hypercalcaemia

Excess vitamin D (usually from pharmaceutical vitamin D ingestion but also in cutaneous sarcoidosis) can give rise to hypercalcaemia with symptoms of lethargy, bone pain, polyuria, constipation, dehydration and renal stones. In this circumstance the circulating level of PTH is suppressed. However, the commonest cause of hypercalcaemia is due to primary hyperparathyroidism, with PTH being secreted from a parathyroid adenoma. In this circumstance serum PTH will be normal or elevated. This may also give rise to 'brown tumours' in bone. Hypercalcaemia of malignancy is usually due to the secretion of tumoural parathormone related peptide (PTHrP) which elevates the calcium and thus suppresses PTH.

Hypercalcaemia >3.0 mmol/l is usually a medical emergency and requires adequate fluid resuscitation with intravenous fluids. A sample for PTH must be taken before treatment is commenced to avoid difficulty in diagnosis later. Further therapy may include bisphosphonate infusions.

Osteoporosis

Osteoporosis is common, is a major public health issue and may be defined as a reduction in bone mass and disruption of cancellous bone structure leading to increased fracture risk. Bone is progressively lost in both sexes from early middle age, but osteoporosis is far more prevalent in postmenopausal women due to oestrogen deficiency. There are as yet unidentified genetic risk factors for osteoporosis. An incomplete list of risk factors include oestrogen and testosterone deficiency (of any cause) in women and men respectively, glucocorticoid use, hyperparathyroidism, malabsorption, renal tubular acidosis, thyrotoxicosis, and Cushing's syndrome. Serum calcium is normal.

Assessment is made by bone densitometry. Treatment is directed at correcting any underlying cause, hormone replacement therapy, calcium and vitamin D supplements, and bisphosphonates.

Pituitary disease

Pituitary disease manifests either through the local symptoms caused by expansion of a pituitary tumour within the confines of the sella, or due to either the excessive secretion of pituitary hormone, or deficiency of pituitary hormone. A large expanding pituitary tumour may cause optic chiasmal compression with associated visual field defects and there may also be headaches.

A pituitary macroadenoma may cause expansion of the pituitary fossa and erosion of the sella turcica. The expansion is frequently asymmetrical and on a true lateral skull radiograph taken in the exact horizontal plane (with both anterior clinoid processes in alignment) this process may give rise to the classic appearance of a double floor sella. If, however, the radiograph is taken with any degree of head tilt then a double-floored fossa will be seen in normal individuals. A lateral skull X-ray as a primary investigation for pituitary disease is obsolete.

Acromegaly

Excessive growth hormone (GH) secretion from a pituitary tumour causes acromegaly with associated bony overgrowth in adults and gigantism in children. There is also an increase in soft tissue, swelling and sweatiness of the hands. Excess GH gives rise to the characteristic 'spade-like' hands, frontal bossing, prognathism, interdental separation, dental malocclusion, macroglossia, hypertension, diabetes mellitus, cardiomyopathy and multinodular goitre (see Colour Plate 19).

Acromegaly is rare (incidence 1:100,000) but requires a high index of suspicion to consider the diagnosis, as the onset is often insidious over many years. Confirmation of the diagnosis is achieved biochemically, with failure of suppression of growth hormone on a glucose tolerance test. The IGF1 level will also be elevated. Referral to an endocrinologist is the appropriate course of action.

Cushing's syndrome

Cushing's syndrome is due to the effects of chronic glucocorticoid excess, most commonly through their use for inflammatory conditions. Endogenous Cushing's syndrome due to excessive cortisol secretion may be due to an adrenal tumour or due to the excessive secretion of ACTH from a pituitary tumour or from an ectopic site such as a lung carcinoid tumour driving the adrenal glands. The commonest cause of this rare condition is a pituitary microadenoma which can only be seen in 50% of cases even with the most sophisticated magnetic resonance imaging (MRI).

The symptoms and signs of this condition are myriad. Classically there is truncal obesity, proximal muscle wasting and myopathy, thin skin, easy bruising, violaceous striae on the trunk, interscapular fat pad (the so-called Buffalo hump), depression, amenorrhoea, osteoporosis, acne, hirsutism, hypertension, diabetes mellitus, and, in children, decreased linear growth. The difficulty is that many of these features are present in other conditions such as depression and the polycystic ovarian syndrome, both of which are common. Biochemical confirmation is mandatory but complex and beyond the scope of this chapter. If suspected referral to an endocrinologist is appropriate.

Hypopituitarism

Hypopituitarism – either due to a pituitary tumour or following pituitary surgery or radiotherapy – results in the patient being on replacement therapy. The most important replacement therapy is hydrocortisone as this is effectively metabolised to cortisol and forms the body's major glucocorticoid. The normal individual's response to stress is a rapid rise in the level of cortisol, and this is required to maintain vascular tone and prevent cardiovascular collapse (Figure 6.2). Individuals with hypopituitarism are unable to respond in this way and therefore require glucocorticoid cover for anything but the most minor of procedures.

For simple dental procedures, the patient should be advised to double their dose of hydrocortisone on the day before, the day of and

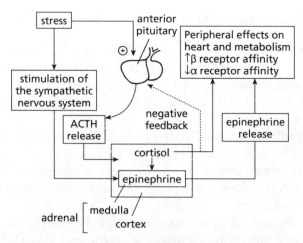

Figure 6.2 The effects of stress on the adrenal production of cortisol and epinephrine (adrenaline).

the day after the procedure. For more complex procedures not requiring general anaesthesia, the patient should be given parenteral hydrocortisone 100 mg intramuscularly at the onset of the procedure, which will give them effective cover for a six-hour period. In addition to this they should 'double up' on their hydrocortisone as indicated above. If there is any doubt, the advice of an endocrinologist should be sought. For general anaesthesia cover should be given as hydrocortisone 100 mg IM with premed and then strictly six-hourly until eating and drinking.

Adrenal disease and steroid therapy

Adrenal failure may be due to either autoimmune Addison's disease or infiltration by tuberculosis, and much less commonly due to metastatic replacement of adrenal tissue. The adrenals produce adrenaline (epinephrine) in addition to cortisol, and are involved in the reaction to 'stress' (Figure 6.2).

Patients on long-term glucocorticoid and mineralocorticoid therapy should be treated in the same way as indicated above for pituitary patients on glucocorticoid replacement therapy. Young patients with hypertension, especially if there is a history of palpitations, should be considered for referral to an endocrinologist to exclude phaeochromocytoma. Operative intervention on these patients may induce a hypertensive crisis with a high level of mortality.

Patients on long-term glucocorticoids, such as prednisolone for lung disease and other inflammatory conditions, will be adrenally suppressed if the daily dose of prednisolone is >7.5 mg/day. These patients should be managed as if hypopituitary (see above).

Summary: Endocrine diseases

- **Hyperthyroidism** is commonly due to three causes: Graves' disease, an autoimmune condition with hyperthyroidism stimulated by circulating immunoglobulins, toxic multinodular goitre and toxic adenoma. All will exhibit a suppressed TSH with elevated levels of free T_3 and free T_4.
- **Hypothyroidism** is usually due to autoimmune thyroid destruction. When untreated, the TSH will be elevated.
- **Severe hypercalcaemia** is a medical emergency warranting immediate referral for treatment. The commonest cause is primary hyperparathyroidism.
- **Pituitary disease** can present due to local features on expanding pituitary mass, hormone excess, e.g. acromegaly with bony overgrowth, or hormone deficiency, in particular glucocorticoid deficiency requiring replacement therapy and cover for surgical procedures.
- **Adrenal disease**: Patients with adrenal failure or on long-term steroid treatment will require hydrocortisone cover for surgical procedures.

Diabetes mellitus

Diabetes mellitus is a metabolic disorder caused by an absolute or relative deficiency of insulin which results in chronic hyperglycaemia. It affects at least 2% of the UK population and the worldwide prevalence is expected to double over the next 20 years. The effects of hyperglycaemia often lead to an increased susceptibility to oral pathology. Diabetes is, therefore, commonly met in routine dental practice and it is vital that dentists understand how their practice affects diabetes.

Insulin

Insulin is the key hormone involved in the storage and controlled release within the body of chemical energy available from food. It is an anabolic hormone. It facilitates the uptake of glucose into muscle and adipose tissue leading to storage of fat and protein. It also regulates hepatic glucose metabolism by increasing glycogen synthesis from glucose and reducing gluconeogenesis.

Insulin deficiency leads to a catabolic state. Glucose uptake into muscle and adipose tissue is reduced and muscle and adipose tissue are broken down. In the liver glycogen is broken down, glucose synthesis is increased and fatty acids are converted into ketones. This process results in hyperglycaemia and if there is an absolute

Table 6.1 Clinical features of type 1 and type 2 diabetes

Type 1 diabetes	Type 2 diabetes
absolute insulin deficiency	relative insulin deficiency/resistance
prone to ketosis	not prone to ketosis
insulin treatment mandatory	diet, tablets or insulin treatment

deficiency of insulin (as in type 1 diabetes), ketosis and a metabolic acidosis.

Diabetes classification

Diabetes mellitus is diagnosed on a random venous glucose concentration of 11.1 mmol/l or greater or fasting plasma glucose of 7.0 mmol/l or greater. In the absence of symptoms of hyperglycaemia diagnosis should not be based on a single glucose determination. Primary diabetes may be classified simply into two main syndromes: type 1 diabetes and type 2 diabetes (Table 6.1).

From a practical point of view the main difference is that type 1 diabetes is caused by an absolute deficiency of insulin, insulin treatment is mandatory and without exogenous insulin ketosis will occur. Type 2 diabetes is due to a relative deficiency of insulin due to insulin resistance and rarely causes ketosis.

Consequences of hyperglycaemia

The consequences of hyperglycaemia are similar in both type 1 and type 2 diabetes, namely: hyperglycaemia, microvascular damage and macrovascular damage.

Hyperglycaemia

Blood glucose levels exceeding the usual renal threshold of 10 mmol/l lead to an osmotic diuresis. This is responsible for the typical symptoms of diabetes: polyuria, thirst and polydipsia. The ensuing catabolic state is associated with fatigue and in type 1 diabetic patients weight loss.

Microvascular damage

Microvascular damage is specific to diabetes. Small blood vessels throughout the body are affected, but the disease process has specific effects in three particular sites: the retina, the renal glomerulus and the nerve. The consequences of microvascular damage at these sites are progressive retinal damage and potential blindness, renal failure and diabetic neuropathy (which increases the risk of foot ulceration).

Macrovascular damage

People with diabetes have between two and three times increased risk of macrovascular complications compared with the general population. This is manifest by an increased prevalence of ischaemic heart disease, peripheral vascular disease and cerebrovascular accident.

Treatment

Type 1 diabetes: Patients with type 1 diabetes have an absolute requirement for insulin which they must inject between two and five times daily. Patients usually check their blood sugar frequently in order to adjust the insulin dose to account for dietary variation and exercise. Insulin may be simply classified into two types: unmodified, quick acting insulin (the patient may refer to this as 'clear' insulin) which is injected prior to meals, and modified or delayed action insulin which is injected once or twice daily to ensure a continuous background insulin.

Type 2 diabetes: Patients with type 2 diabetes may be managed by dietary restriction alone, with diet and oral hypoglycaemics or diet in combination with insulin.

Diabetic problems of relevance to the dentist

Stress

The usual balance between anabolism and catabolism is disrupted during metabolic stress such as infection, intercurrent illness or surgery. Insulin deficiency exaggerates this imbalance further in favour of increased catabolism. Metabolic stress results in reduced insulin action which causes hyperglycaemia, protein loss and ketosis (Figure 6.3).

In type 1 diabetes metabolic stress may lead to diabetic ketoacidotic coma if the amount injected is not increased. Patients with type 2 diabetes have endogenous insulin production and are not prone to ketoacidosis. They are, however, prone to hyperglycaemia and consequent dehydration and may also need to increase hypoglycaemic treatment.

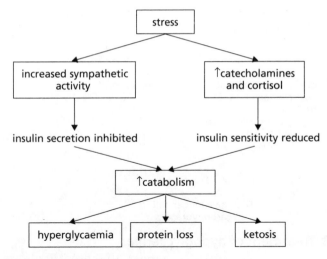

Figure 6.3 The metabolic response to stress.

Hypoglycaemia

Hypoglycaemia occurs when hepatic glucose output falls below the rate of glucose uptake by peripheral tissues. In practice a blood sugar of less than 4 mmol/l is considered abnormally low, and symptoms of hypoglycaemia become evident as the blood sugar falls to around 3 mmol/l. Symptoms of hypoglycaemia can be classified into those caused by autonomic activation and those caused by neuroglyco-penia, as follows:

Autonomic activation:

- sweating
- tremor
- palpitation
- blurred vision
- headache

Neuroglycopenia:

- cognitive impairment
- drowsiness
- inco-ordination
- confusion
- coma
- fits

Patients with diabetes are usually able to recognise hypoglycaemic symptoms and treat hypoglycaemia with extra carbohydrate. In

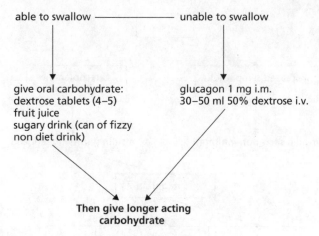

able to swallow ——————— unable to swallow

give oral carbohydrate:
dextrose tablets (4–5)
fruit juice
sugary drink (can of fizzy
non diet drink)

glucagon 1 mg i.m.
30–50 ml 50% dextrose i.v.

**Then give longer acting
carbohydrate**

Figure 6.4 Treatment of hypoglycaemia.

some patients, however, adrenergic symptoms of hypoglycaemia are reduced or absent and they have to rely on the more subjective neuroglycopenic symptoms which may not occur until blood sugars fall below 2 mmol/l. This increases the risk of hypoglycaemia going unnoticed until severe hypoglycaemia ensues and possible coma.

In dental practice the risk of hypoglycaemia can be reduced by ensuring dental treatment does not interfere with eating and normal meal times. If hypoglycaemia occurs it may be treated as detailed in Figure 6.4.

Summary: Management of problems in diabetics

• **Hypoglycaemia**: Avoid disruption to usual eating patterns. Plan treatment for just after breakfast and usual hypoglycaemic medication for procedures under local anaesthetic. If difficulty with normal eating after procedure is expected, discuss management with diabetic patient's physician and consider referral to hospital.
• **Dental infection/risk of ketosis**: Patients on insulin should increase blood sugar monitoring and increase insulin doses as appropriate. Patients unable to do this should be referred to diabetes team for advice.
• **Need for general anaesthesia/sedation**: These patients should always be referred to hospital for specialist care. Local guidelines for management of diabetic patients undergoing day patient procedures should be followed. In practice, well-controlled patients, without complications undergoing short procedures (<60 minutes) are suitable for day case procedures.

Tiredness

Many patients will mention tiredness as a secondary problem, even when it is not a presenting symptom. The physician's role is to identify if any serious medical problem underlies the complaint. A recent survey of patients attending my outpatient clinic with a wide range of medical complaints showed that only 9% of them described themselves as having 'normal energy', 27% as 'so-so', 54% were 'often tired', 9% were 'always tired' and 0% 'full of energy'! Tiredness, for whatever reason, and to varying degrees of severity, is a problem for a considerable proportion of people, or at least those who attend hospital medical clinics.

For many people tiredness can clearly be pinpointed as having an underlying social, rather than medical cause – e.g. pressures of family responsibilities, overwhelming occupational duties, excessive participation in social activities. It generally reflects that patients overestimate their own physical abilities to cope with demanding lifestyles. However, tiredness may also be a presenting symptom for a number of serious medical conditions which require investigation and treatment. These include:

• **Depression**: A positive additional history may be obtained of poor appetite, poor sleeping pattern, weepiness, loss of interest in daily activities and previous depressive illness.

• **Haematological disorders**, particularly iron deficiency anaemia if it is severe enough. A cause for the iron deficiency needs to be identified from: oesophageal disease, peptic ulcer disease, gastric tumour, large bowel tumour, inflammatory bowel disease, diverticulosis, malabsorption, hypernephroma or bladder cancer, menorrhagia (including fibroid, tumour or hypothyroidism).

• **Infective disorders**: Other symptoms such as fever and symptoms localised to the specific systems involved by the infection are likely to provide the presenting complaint but tiredness is relevant in subacute or chronic infective states, particularly: postviral including 'ME' and, very importantly, infectious mononucleosis, subacute bacterial endocarditis and tuberculosis.

• **Chronic renal failure**: Patients with this can be anaemic.

• **Congestive cardiac failure**, although in this case other symptoms are probably of greater significance, especially breathlessness and oedema.

Weight loss

Unintended weight loss is a symptom of extreme importance in the medical history, particularly when it has been clearly documented and is sudden and rapid in nature. The physician ignores significant weight loss at both their own and the patient's peril. The age of the patient may be of significance, particularly when considering the possibility of an underlying cancer and, in younger people, other problems, including endocrine, psychiatric and infective disorders should be considered. Significant problems to be considered here include:

- **Depression**: Depressed patients can have significant somatic signs.
- **Anorexia nervosa**: Other evidence for the disorder will need to be looked for, including dental evidence, lanugo hairs and amenorrhoea. Of course, the patient themselves may not necessarily be complaining of weight loss.
- **Endocrine disorders**: Diabetes mellitus, hyperthyroidism, hypopituitarism, and Addison's disease.
- **Cancer**: Weight loss is frequently an important manifestation of a broad range of neoplasms either as the sole presenting symptom or in association with other symptoms. Consider particularly carcinomas of the stomach, bronchus, oesophagus, large bowel, pancreas and kidney.
- **Other gastroenterological disorders** including malabsorption due to coeliac disease and inflammatory bowel.
- **Other chronic or subacute disorders**: Similar to the list for 'Tiredness' including infective (e.g. tuberculosis, or postviral, especially infectious mononucleosis) and chronic renal failure.
- **Weight varies throughout life**: As people move from middle age to old age, muscle bulk and body fat is reduced and weight loss to some degree is quite normal. A balance must therefore be struck when considering the investigation of say, a 70-year-old who has lost half a stone in weight in the past six months and in deciding to what extent, including using uncomfortable and sometimes invasive procedures, they should be investigated. Evidence provided by other simple tests for anaemia or abnormal liver function may support more detailed, demanding and costly investigations.

Treatment

If these problems are attributable to underlying medical or psychiatric conditions then treatment is clearly centred around dealing with the underlying illness. People with serious illness who have lost weight may require dietary assessment by a dietician who advises on dietary supplementation. Some conditions such as diabetes or coeliac disease will require adjustments to diet which will, in themselves, correct or markedly benefit the illness. Severely ill people may require treatment with parenteral nutrition.

Those without identifiable underlying disease need to be told that there is not a serious problem, and asked to consider alterations to their lifestyle such as reducing family responsibilities, social commitments or hours of work for instance. Most are reassured when all tests are normal and the physician offers such an explanation. A small minority may not be satisfied. For them there may be a role for 'alternative therapies' and support groups.

Summary: Tiredness and weight loss are important medical complaints that may be the presenting symptoms for serious underlying conditions.

- **Tiredness** can be due to depression, blood disorders, endocrine disease, infections and postinfective syndromes, renal failure and heart failure.
- **Weight loss** may be the result of depression, anorexia nervosa, endocrine disease, gastrointestinal disorder, infection and cancer, but in some cases it is due to 'normal' variations seen in the different stages of life.

Further reading

Davey, P. (ed) (2002) *Medicine at a Glance*. Oxford, Blackwell Science.

Grossman, A.B. (ed) (1998) *Clinical Endocrinology*. Oxford, Blackwell Science.

Holmes, S., Alexander, W. (1997) Diabetes in dentistry. *Practical Diabetes*, 14:107–10.

Newell-Price, J.D.C., Grossman, A.B. (1999) The diagnosis and management of Cushing's syndrome. *Lancet*, 353: 2087–8.

Trainer, P.J., Newell-Price, J.D.C., Besser, G.M. Cushing's syndrome. In Wass, J.A., Shalet, S.M. (eds) (2002) *Oxford Textbook of Endocrinology*. Oxford: Oxford University Press.

Websites

Endocrine Society: http://www.endo-society.org

Diabetes overview:
   http://www.niddk.nih.gov/health/diabetes/pubs/dmover/dmover.htm

Unintentional weight loss:
   http://health.yahoo.com/health/encyclopedia/003107/0.html

CHAPTER 7
Renal Diseases

The kidneys are located behind the peritoneum, high in the posterior abdomen (Figure 7.1). Their function is to excrete the waste products of metabolism, regulate total body water, electrolyte and acid-base balance, to produce certain hormones (e.g. erythropoietin for red blood cell regulation, 1,25-dihydroxy vitamin D for calcium metabolism, and renin/angiotensin for electrolyte balance), and to excrete water-soluble drugs. The most common renal problems

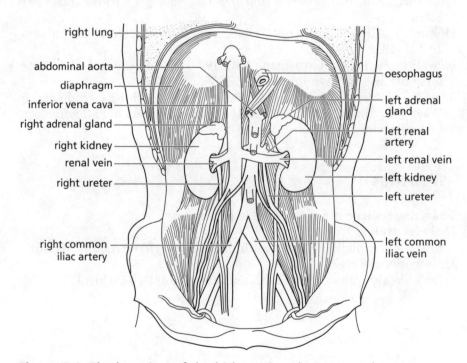

right lung
abdominal aorta
diaphragm
inferior vena cava
right adrenal gland
right kidney
renal vein
right ureter
right common iliac artery

oesophagus
left adrenal gland
left renal artery
left renal vein
left kidney
left ureter
left common iliac vein

Figure 7.1 The location of the kidneys in relation to other structures in the upper abdomen.

that the dentist is likely to encounter are renal failure and renal transplant.

Renal failure

Renal failure can be either acute or chronic. Acute renal failure (ARF) is usually of sudden onset, short duration and is reversible within six to eight weeks. The major causes of ARF can be divided into pre-renal, renal and post-renal.

Pre-renal refers to any haemodynamic cause jeopardising renal perfusion such as hypovolaemia and hypotension. Renal denotes causes of intrinsic renal disease such as an acute inflammation of the glomeruli (glomerulonephritis), of the tubulointerstitium (acute interstitial nephritis), hypertensive crisis (accelerated hypertension) or direct damage to the kidneys caused by drugs or toxins. Post-renal ARF refers to all the causes related to an obstruction of the urinary flow distal to the kidneys. These could include renal stones, tumours, clots or fibrosis.

Chronic renal failure (CRF) is defined as a longstanding and usually irreversible cause of renal insufficiency. The severity of CRF can be classified as shown in Table 7.1.

Incidence and prevalence

The incidence of end-stage renal failure (ESRF) in the UK is around 100 new patients per million of population (pmp) per year. This leads to a prevalence of patients receiving renal replacement therapy (dialysis/transplantation) of around 300–400 pmp. The incidence and prevalence of ESRF in the UK is lower than in Europe and much lower than in the US where they reach 290 pmp/year and 900 pmp respectively. This may be due to differences in the populations' profile and ethnicity but also to the limitation of resources in the UK. The prevalence of ESRF clearly reflects a higher prevalence of CRF in the population, estimated by some to be as high as 2000 pmp.

Table 7.1 Classification of the severity of chronic renal failure

Severity	Glomerular filtration rate (GFR) (ml/min)	Serum creatinine (µmol/l)
Normal range	100–120	~80–100
Mild	90–50	~80–100
Moderate	49–25	~120–200
Severe	24–10	~200–600
Endstage	<10	>600–1000

Causes of chronic renal failure

There are several causes of CRF. They are listed in order of frequency:
• **chronic glomerulonephritis**: inflammation of the glomeruli
• **hypertension**: damages kidney vessels and function
• **diabetes**: affects glomerular capillaries
• **interstitial nephritis**: includes recurrent infections and drugs exposure
• **polycystic kidney disease**: inherited degenerative condition.

Clinical presentation

Patients with underlying renal diseases can present to medical attention in one of many ways. It may occur as an incidental finding, e.g. from hypertension, abnormal serum creatinine, haematuria or proteinuria, or due to symptomatic disease, e.g. haematuria, urinary tract infections, pain over kidneys, or symptoms related to hypertension, proteinuria (oedema) or renal insufficiency.

The symptoms of severe renal insufficiency (uraemia) develop insidiously and late. Uraemic symptoms do not usually appear until the patient's GFR is less than 20 ml/minute. The most common uraemic symptoms are fatigue, nausea and vomiting, anorexia, ankle swelling, itching, muscle cramps and the inability to concentrate.

History

A careful medical history should attempt to define:
• the **cause of renal disease**, including a thorough family history
• **predisposing factors** such as diabetes, hypertension, urinary tract infections, medication including chronic abuse of analgesics and non-steroidals and exposure to toxins
• **family history** of hereditary renal disorders, diabetes or hypertension
• **manifestations of renal diseases**: haematuria, hypertension, oedema, nocturia, dysuria, frequency, pregnancy-related hypertension or proteinuria
• **complications of renal diseases**: cardiovascular, anaemia, musculoskeletal, gastrointestinal.

Physical signs of renal failure

Physical signs should focus on signs that point to the cause of renal failure, its chronicity and its complications:

Signs pointing to the underlying disease

- **diabetes mellitus**: diabetic retinopathy and neuropathy
- **hypertension**: hypertensive retinopathy
- **polycystic kidney disease**: large cystic kidneys

Signs reflecting chronicity of renal disease

- **anaemia**: pallor
- **skin**: yellow-brown discoloration, nail dystrophy, ecchymoses
- **hypertension**: cardiomegaly, congestive heart failure, hypertensive retinopathy

Signs of uraemic complications

- **anaemia**: pallor
- **cutaneous**: yellow-brown discoloration
- **bleeding tendency**: ecchymoses, purpura (see Colour Plate 5)
- **Cardiovascular**: cardiomegaly and heart failure
- **valvular calcifications**: valvular stenosis/regurgitation, heart murmurs
- **ocular**: hypertensive retinopathy
- **immunosuppression**: infections
- **neurological**: peripheral neuropathy

Laboratory investigations in chronic renal failure

The full blood count shows a low haemoglobin, but a normal white cell and platelet count. In the coagulation screen, the prothrombin and partial thromboplastin times are normal but the bleeding time is prolonged and the erythrocyte sedimentation rate is high. Serum biochemical tests reveal an elevation of the urea and creatinine, a low or normal sodium, a high potassium, a low bicarbonate and calcium, and a high phosphate. The 24-hour urinary protein is high (>300 mg/24h) and the creatinine clearance is reduced.

Systemic complications of CRF with relevance to dentists

Cardiovascular

There are three cardiovascular problems of relevance to the dentist: hypertension, congestive heart failure, and calcification of the heart valves.

Homeostasis

Potential clotting includes thrombocytopenia (rare), a bleeding tendency, and a prolonged bleeding time due to platelet dysfunction. A more common problem is the effect of uraemic toxins on platelet function, particularly adhesion and aggregation. This may exacerbate uraemic anaemia and renal osteodystrophy. Lack of activated vitamin D results in osteomalacia, excessive parathyroid hormone in osteitis fibrosa, and mixed renal osteodystrophy in osteosclerosis, which affects the bones of the jaw with subperiosteal resorption.

Immunosuppression

Uraemia tends to lead to immunosuppression and susceptibility to infections. Peridontitis is common. The treatment of the majority of glomerulonephritides consists of immunosuppression with steroids and/or other immunosuppressive agents.

Management of chronic renal failure

Management of the underlying disease

- **glomerulonephritis**: immunosuppression
- **hypertension**: blood pressure control
- **diabetes**: glycaemic control
- **recurrent UTI**: antibiotics

Management of uraemic complications

- **anaemia**: iron and erythropoietin
- **hypertension**: antihypertensives
- **renal osteodystrophy**: calcium and vitamin D
- **undernutrition**: caloric supplementation and vitamins
  Also attention should be paid to avoid nephrotoxins: e.g. non-steroidal anti-inflammatory drugs are potentially nephrotoxic, as are angiotensin converting enzyme inhibitors. The metabolism and clearance of many drugs are affected by renal failure, e.g. opiates accumulate, cause drowsiness and even stupor or coma.

Dialysis replacement therapy

When renal function reaches end stage and the GFR is less than 10 ml/min, patients are started on one of two renal replacement therapy options: haemodialysis (HD) and continuous ambulatory peritoneal dialysis (CAPD).

Haemodialysis

HD consists of the purification of the patient's blood through an extra-corporeal system including the dialysis (filter). On average patients dialyse thrice weekly for four hours a time. Haemodialysis patients are heparinised during the dialysis session.

Complications of haemodialysis include:
- **bleeding tendency** worsens
- **uraemic complications** progress
- high morbidity and mortality from **cardiovascular complications** including ischaemic heart disease and strokes
- **renal osteodystrophy** worsens
- increased **susceptibility to infection**
- increased incidence of **peridontitis**
- chronic infections contribute to **malnutrition, morbidity and mortality**
- increased incidence of **malignancy**.

Continuous ambulatory peritoneal dialysis

Same complications as with HD. In addition, tendency to hypo-albuminaemia and wasting. Less bleeding tendency as the patients do not receive anticoagulants.

The presence of an indwelling peritoneal catheter does not constitute an indication for prophylactic antibiotics in relation to dental work.

Renal transplantation

Three type of transplant donors are contemplated: cadaveric, live-related and live-unrelated. The **complications** of renal transplantation are as follows:
- **renal**: recurrence of the original nephropathy, acute rejection, chronic allograft nephropathy and hypertension
- **related to immunosuppression**: susceptibility to infections, opportunistic infections and malignancy
- **drug-related**: e.g. the effects of steroids, azathioprine, or cyclosporin (including gingival hypertrophy).

Summary: Renal diseases

Patients with underlying renal diseases and renal insufficiency are at increased risk of:

- **Cardiovascular disease** including systemic hypertension and ischaemic heart disease.
- **Valvular heart disease** as uraemic patients develop metastatic calcifications including aortic and mitral calcifications.
- **Infectious complications** due to uraemic immunosuppression and the effects of drugs used to treat their underlying disease or to induce tolerance after transplantation.
- **Malnutrition** due to a combination of anorexia and hypercatabolism.
- **Bleeding tendency** due to uraemic platelet dysfunction and to the effects of anticoagulation for patients treated by haemodialysis.

Further reading

El Nahas, A.M., Winearls, C.G. (1996) Chronic renal failure. In Weatherall, D.J., Ledingham, J.G.G., Warrell, D.A. (eds) *Oxford Textbook of Medicine.* Oxford, Oxford University Press, Vol 3, pp. 3294–305.

El Nahas, A.M. (2000) Progression of chronic renal failure. In Johnson, R.J. and Feehally, J. (eds) *Comprehensive Clinical Nephrology.* London, Mosby, 2000, pp. 67.1–10.

Winearls, C.G. (2000) Clinical evaluation and manifestations of chronic renal failure. In Johnson, R.J. and Feehally, J. (eds) *Comprehensive Clinical Nephrology.* London, Mosby, pp. 68.1–14.

Website

Sheffield Kidney Institute: http://www.shef.ac.uk/ski/

CHAPTER 8
Neurological Diseases

Many neurological disorders are common and the dentist is required to know whether any special precautions are needed in patients with these conditions or on medication for them. In addition, patients may present to the dentist with neurological symptoms or signs on the face that may be the presenting feature of a neurological condition. Some of the most important neurological complaints are described in this section.

Multiple sclerosis

Multiple sclerosis (MS) is a chronic disorder in which episodes of demyelination affect any part of the central nervous system producing a multiplicity of symptoms and signs. It often begins with a relapsing and remitting course, which eventually culminates in a progressive phase with a gradual accumulation of wide-ranging disabilities. In the UK, the prevalence is about 100 per 100,000. Symptoms and signs depend on the site of pathology and include:
- **optic nerve**: attacks of retro-orbital pain, blurred vision, reduced visual acuity, and central scotoma
- **brain stem**: diplopia, dysconjugate eye movements, dysarthria, vertigo, ataxia, and tremor
- **spinal cord**: sensory symptoms, spastic weakness, and bladder/bowel/sexual dysfunction
- **trigeminal neuralgia-like facial pain**: some 2–3% of patients with trigeminal neuralgia have MS. This can occasionally be the first manifestation of MS and should always be considered when patients under the age of 50 present with trigeminal neuralgia
- **others**: euphoria, dementia, and painful tonic spasms.

MS is a clinical diagnosis and no test is pathognomonic. However, magnetic resonance imaging (MRI) of the brain and spinal cord shows areas of abnormal signal in the white matter in almost all patients. Acute relapses are treated with oral or intravenous steroids. Interferon-beta and glatiramer acetate are effective in reducing relapse rate and disease progression. No special considerations are needed in most patients with MS who attend for dental treatment.

Epilepsy

An epileptic seizure (fit) is a paroxysmal alteration in nervous system activity that is time limited and causes a clinically detectable event. Epilepsy is a condition in which more than one seizure has occurred. Epileptic seizures can be focal (simple or complex) or generalised (absence, tonic–clonic, myoclonic, or atonic). A patient who has had a seizure with loss of consciousness may remember feeling odd (e.g. odd smells, metallic taste) before the event (the aura) and may remain confused and disorientated afterwards (the postictal phase) but will have no memory of the fit itself. Tongue biting and urinary incontinence are frequently seen.

Epilepsy is a clinical diagnosis and patients are often normal on examination. An eyewitness account is vital in establishing the diagnosis. Investigations include computed tomography (CT) or MRI scans to rule out the presence of any focal brain pathology (e.g. a tumour or a stroke). An electroencephalogram (EEG) is usually performed. This is frequently normal and this does not disprove the diagnosis. There is a wide range of anti-epileptic medications and the choice depends mostly on seizure type. Factors that could induce seizures include sleep depravation, alcohol, antiepileptic medications withdrawal and intercurrent illnesses.

Dental treatment in a patient with controlled epilepsy can proceed as normal but the dentist should be aware of how to deal with a fit were it to occur.

Cerebrovascular disease

The brain has a rich blood supply derived from the internal carotid and vertebral arteries. Stroke is a focal neurological deficit of a presumed vascular origin. Thromboembolic infarctions constitute about 85% of all strokes. Haemorrhagic strokes are less frequent (15%). The clinical features are extremely variable and depend on the site and the extent of the lesion.

Transient ischaemic attacks (TIA) often herald completed strokes and should therefore be investigated promptly. Skilled nursing and physiotherapy are the main pillars of treatment. For secondary prevention all risk factors (hypertension, diabetes, smoking, hyperlipidaemia, cardiac arrhythmias) should be modified. Anti-platelet drugs such as aspirin, and endarterectomy, should be considered.

Patients who have had a stroke may have a disability that affects the practical administration of their dental treatment (see Chapter 19).

Headache

Headache is a frequent symptom and often due to stress. Investigations are rarely needed. The main decision in the clinical approach to headache is to ascertain whether the headache is a new event or one of a recurrent series. As a general rule one should consider the possibility of an underlying neurological illness if the headache is a new event in a subject who never suffered from headaches before.

Acute single episodes: When headache is generalised and associated with drowsiness and neck stiffness **meningitis** and **encephalitis** should be excluded. **Subarachnoid haemorrhage** usually presents with a sudden severe headache associated with nausea, photophobia, drowsiness and neck stiffness. **Sinusitis** may also present as an acute unilateral frontomaxillary pain associated with local tenderness.

Acute recurrent episodes: **Migraine** is the commonest cause. Episodes often begin with visual aura (scintillating scotomas, flickering lights) followed some 10–60 minutes later by a unilateral throbbing headache with nausea, vomiting, photophobia, and phonophobia. **Cluster headache** presents as daily headache that lasts a few weeks and comes in clusters every few weeks. Episodes start at night as severe unilateral peri-orbital pain often associated with lacrimation and rhinorrhoea and last up to an hour at a time.

Subacute headaches: In patients over 55 years, **giant cell arteritis** should be excluded. Patients may report jaw claudication and often have tender, thickened, and pulseless temporal arteries. Erythrocyte sedimentation rate (ESR) is usually high. The condition responds to treatment with steroids.

Chronic headaches: **Tension headache** usually presents as daily, pressure like bitemporal headache which tends to get worse as the day goes on. This headache is often associated with long-term use of analgesics. The headache of **raised intracranial pressure** (space occupying lesions, benign intracranial hypertension) tends to present on waking. It is often accompanied by vomiting and blurred vision, and is made worse by coughing and bending.

Dentists who have a patient who complains of acute recurrent headache should refer them to a general medical practitioner.

Cranial nerve palsies

There are 12 cranial nerves. These nerves contain motor, sensory, or both types of fibre. They emerge from the underside of the brain (Figure 8.1). Some of the cranial nerves are of importance in dentistry because they innervate the tongue, mouth or mandible. All others are of relevance as a dentist may be the first clinician to notice a lesion of a cranial nerve and thereby has a duty of care to make the appropriate referral.

Disorders of the cranial nerves will be dealt with in the numerical order of these nerves, although the cranial nerve problems of relevance to the dentist will mainly be of the trigeminal, facial, glossopharyngeal and hypoglossal nerves.

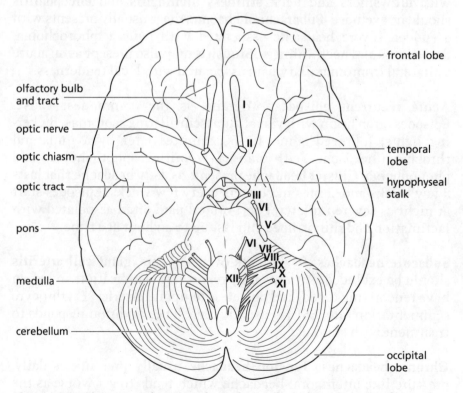

Figure 8.1 The cranial nerves (numbered) as they emerge from the lower surface of the brain.

Olfactory nerve (cranial nerve I)

Loss of smell used to be an important clue to anterior fossa floor tumours in cases of dementia or altered behaviour. It is less important now as these patients are screened by CT scan.

Optic nerve (cranial nerve II)

Damage to the optic nerve causes monocular visual loss, optic atrophy (which takes several months to develop) and a Marcus Gunn pupil (when a light is swung from the good to the bad eye the pupil of the bad eye dilates).

Oculomotor nerve (cranial nerve III)

The oculomotor nerve innervates most of the muscles of the eye and the striated part of the lid levator muscle. The other outer part is smooth muscle that is innervated by the sympathetic system (hence the development of ptosis in Horner's syndrome). It has a parasympathetic part to the pupil on the upper nerve surface which tends to be involved when masses press on the nerve from outside and spared when the nerve is affected by microvascular disease. For this reason a medical third nerve palsy usually spares the pupil (diabetes is the commonest cause) and a surgical palsy (posterior communicating artery aneurysms or tumours) involves the pupil. A third nerve palsy with headache suggests a posterior communicating artery aneurysm and should be regarded as an emergency.

Trochlear nerve (cranial nerve IV)

The trochlear nerve supplies the superior oblique muscle of the eye. This muscle works with the inferior oblique (oculomotor nerve) to rotate the eye around a horizontal forward pointing axis. Its main effect is to compensate for the secondary rotational effects of the other muscles.

A fourth nerve palsy is very difficult to detect by looking at the eyes in different positions. The clue to a fourth nerve palsy is diplopia where the two images the patient sees are not parallel. The diplopia is worst on looking down and laterally on the affected side.

Trigeminal nerve (cranial nerve V)

Trigeminal neuralgia may be caused by demyelination of the root entry zone of the sensory part of the trigeminal nerve. The commonest cause of this is compression from an anatomical variant of the cerebral artery. Other causes are MS and tumours in the cerebellopontine angle. Treatment is either medical or surgical. Medical consists of carbamazepine as the first line drug. If carbamazepine is ineffective, a second line drug such as phenytoin, lamotrigene or gabapentin is added. Surgical treatment is by surgical nerve injury or decompression by dissecting the vessel off the nerve.

The trigeminal nerve also has a motor function in that it innervates the muscles of mastication, tensor veli palatini, mylohyoid and the anterior belly of the digastric muscle. It causes the 'jaw jerk'.

Abducens nerve (cranial nerve VI)

The abducens nerve supplies the lateral rectus muscle of the eye. It is frequently involved in intracranial disease. A sixth nerve palsy means the affected eye cannot abduct. Paresis leads to diplopia with parallel images.

Facial nerve (cranial nerve VII)

A motor palsy of the facial nerve is known as a Bell's palsy (see Colour Plate 23). It is characterised by a spontaneous lower motor neuron type facial weakness of rapid onset and is possibly of viral aetiology. Recovery is the rule. If the palsy is complete, recovery may be incomplete and steroid treatment may help. A facial nerve palsy may be a sign of a tumour in the parotid gland. If there is a facial weakness then the tumour is probably malignant. The facial nerve also has a sensory function as sensory fibres innervate a small area of the external ear and the anterior two-thirds of the tongue where they are responsible for the sensation of taste (Figure 8.2).

Acoustic nerve (cranial nerve VIII)

Sudden onset sensorineural deafness on one side is usually of viral origin. It may or may not recover. MRI scanning to look for an acoustic 'neuroma' (actually a schwannoma) is recommended in cases of unilateral hearing loss.

Glossopharyngeal nerve (cranial nerve IX)

Only one muscle is supplied by this nerve – the stylopharyngeus. This cannot be tested clinically. It is not the motor supply to the palate (this is supplied by the vagus nerve). The glossopharyngeal nerve supplies sensation to the pharynx and the posterior third of the tongue. It is responsible for taste sensation from the posterior

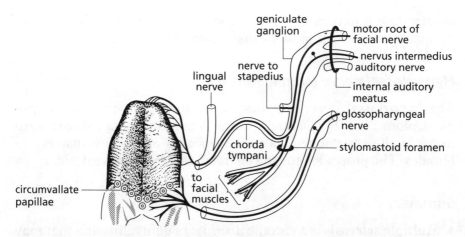

Figure 8.2 The taste pathways of the tongue from the facial and glossopharyngeal nerves and the essential components of the facial nerve.

third of the tongue and for general sensation in the posterior third of the tongue and in the pharynx.

The gag reflex (elevation of soft palate when the back of the throat is prodded) is afferent via the glossopharyngeal nerve and efferent via the vagus. In glossopharyngeal neuralgia, there is lancinating pain that affects the back of the throat. Medical treatment as for trigeminal neuralgia; needle damage to nerve possible. Specialist referral is recommended because of the rarity of the condition.

Vagus nerve (cranial nerve X)

The vagus has both motor and sensory components. The motor innervation is to the palate and vocal cords (recurrent to cords on both sides. The left vagus nerve is closely applied to the aorta and may be damaged by mediastinal disease). The sensory innervation is to the outer ear. The vagus also supplies the parasympathetic fibres to the viscera as far as the splenic flexure of the colon. The vagus is tested by observing the quality of the voice and cough (paralysis of one vocal cord means that the cords cannot be opposed and the cough lacks an explosive start) and symmetrical elevation of the palate on saying 'Ah'.

Accessory nerve (cranial nerve XI)

The accessory nerve is motor to the sternomastoid muscle and to the upper part of the trapezius muscle. After nerve damage these become wasted, although weakness is difficult to detect because of overlapping function of other muscles. The accessory nerves are vulnerable to damage in block dissection of the neck.

Hypoglossal nerve (cranial nerve XII)

The hypoglossal nerve supplies motor innervation to the tongue (see Colour Plate 24). Damage is rare. A neurofibroma of the twelfth nerve is the commonest cause and occurs almost exclusively in females. The protruded tongue deviated towards the weak side.

Summary

- **Multiple sclerosis** is a chronic disorder of demyelination that may affect any part of the central nervous system. It has a relapsing and remitting course and can produce a variety of symptoms including visual disturbance, dysarthria, sensory symptoms, spastic weakness, tremor, bladder dysfunction, and facial pain.
- **Epileptic seizures** are paroxysmal alterations in nervous system activity with a clinically detectable event. Seizures are of various types, e.g. tonic–clonic or absence. The patient may bite their tongue or have incontinence of urine.
- **Stroke** is a focal neurological deficit of presumed vascular origin and can be embolic or less commonly haemorrhagic. Transient ischaemic attacks may precede a stroke.
- **Headache** is a common symptom often due to 'stress'. If of sudden onset it may represent meningitis or subarachnoid haemorrhage. Recurrent headaches may represent migraine especially with visual aura. Chronic headaches can indicate raised intracranial pressure.

Table 8.1 Clinical effects of cranial nerve palsies

No	Cranial nerves	Clinical effect of palsy
I	Olfactory	loss of sense of smell
II	Optic	visual loss, abnormal pupil reflex
III	Oculomotor	ptosis with or without constricted pupil
IV	Trochlear	diplopia
V	Trigeminal	loss of facial sensation (and corneal reflex), neuralgia, weakness of masseter muscles
VI	Abducens	diplopia
VII	Facial	facial muscular weakness, loss of taste
VIII	Acoustic	deafness, tinnitus, dizziness
IX	Glossopharyngeal	sensory loss in tongue and pharynx, neuralgia, loss of gag reflex (motor is via vagus)
X	Vagus	abnormal voice (dysarthria, dysphonia), difficulty swallowing, asymmetry of 'ah' reflex
XI	Accessory	wasting of sternomastoid/trapezius muscles
XII	Hypoglossal	tongue wasted, deviates to side of lesion

- **Cranial nerve palsies**: Details of the clinical features are given in Table 8.1.

Further reading

Marsden, C.D., Fowler, T.J. (1998) *Clinical Neurology*. 2nd edition. Oxford, Arnold.

Trend, P., Swash, M., Kennard, C. (1998) *Neurology*. 2nd edition. Edinburgh, Churchill Livingstone.

Website

National Stroke Association USA: http://www.stroke.org/

CHAPTER 9
Haematological Diseases

Several blood disorders are of importance to the dentist and patients on anticoagulants and drugs for certain haematological diseases need particular management. Oral manifestations of haematological disease and their causes include:

- **infections**: leukaemia, aplastic anaemia
- **mouth ulcers**: neutropenia
- **gum bleeding**: thrombocytopenia
- **cyanosis**: polycythaemia, methaemoglobinaemia
- **gum hypertrophy**: acute monocytic leukaemia
- **angular stomatitis**: iron or vitamin B12 deficiency
- **smooth tongue**: iron or vitamin B12 deficiency
- **tonsillar enlargement**: glandular fever, lymphoma
- **macroglossia**: amyloid

Anaemia

Anaemia is defined as a haemoglobin concentration below the lower limit of normal. It can be due to blood loss (e.g. bleeding from menorrhagia), production failure (e.g. due to deficiency of iron, folic acid or vitamin B12), or due to excessive breakdown of red cells in the circulation (e.g. in autoimmune haemolytic anaemia). In all cases the primary cause for the anaemia should be investigated and appropriately treated. Although blood transfusion can produce immediate benefit, this benefit only lasts for 4–6 weeks so it is essential to correct the underlying problem if possible.

Sickle cell disease

Sickle cell disease is an autosomal recessive condition due to a single point mutation in the beta globin chain of haemoglobin. It affects patients of Afro-Caribbean origin with homozygous patients having sickle cell disease, while heterozygous ones have sickle cell trait. Patients with sickle cell trait are entirely asymptomatic and can have dental work with no problems or precautions. Sickle cell disease patients can have crises if exposed to infections, hypoxia or cold temperature. Sickle cell crises are due to polymerisation of the sickle haemoglobin making the red cells irreversibly deformed; these block the capillaries resulting in tissue necrosis distal to the blockage. During dental surgery these patients must be kept well oxygenated and infections should be treated promptly.

Leukaemia and lymphoma

Leukaemia is a neoplastic condition due to the increase in the number of abnormal clonal white cells in the peripheral blood. Lymphomas are neoplastic proliferations of lymphoid cells and tend to be localised in lymph nodes, although there is overlap between the two conditions. The abnormal cells in leukaemia infiltrate the bone marrow and replace the normal haemopoietic activity resulting in bone marrow failure with anaemia, neutropenia and thrombocytopenia.

Leukaemias can be classified into acute (which are aggressive and invariably fatal in a few weeks if untreated) and chronic (which are more gradual and patients may be asymptomatic and survive for years without treatment). Leukaemias are also classified according to the type of cell they affect. Acute lymphoblastic leukaemia occurs in children and has a good prognosis, although treatment with chemotherapy lasts for two years. Chronic lymphatic leukaemia is a common disease of the elderly and is often asymptomatic.

Lymphomas can be classified into Hodgkin's and non-Hodgkin's (NHL) types. They tend to affect the lymph nodes (see Colour Plate 6) and bone marrow failure is usually a late feature of the disease. Non-Hodgkin's lymphomas are further classified depending on the type of lymphocyte affected i.e. whether B or T and whether mature or immature. Treatment is with either chemotherapy, radiotherapy or both.

Myeloma

Myeloma is a neoplastic disorder of plasma cells, which are terminally differentiated B-lymphocytes. The plasma cell proliferation within the bone marrow leads to lytic lesions and produce monoclonal immunoglobulin, which can be detected in the peripheral blood.

Patients present with bone pain, renal impairment, hypercalcaemia and hyperviscosity. Treatment is with chemotherapy and sometimes radiotherapy, especially for localised disease.

Bleeding disorders

Haemophilia is an inherited sex-linked bleeding disorder found in all populations. Haemophilia A is due to deficiency of Factor VIII and affects 1 in 5000 males, while haemophilia B, which is due to deficiency of Factor IX, is five times rarer. Bleeding is usually into the joints or muscle and patients bleed postoperatively including following dental extractions (Figure 9.1). Patients with severe disease have less than 1% of the normal factor and bleed spontaneously into their joints up to several times per week. Although patients with milder disease do not bleed spontaneously they will bleed after trauma.

Bleeding into a joint is called haemarthrosis and after repeated episodes the synovium lining the joint is damaged leading to chronic crippling arthritis. Once a bleed develops, and prior to surgery,

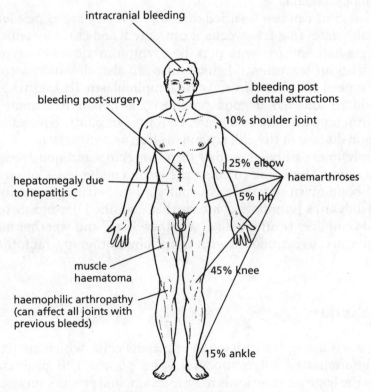

intracranial bleeding

bleeding post-surgery

bleeding post dental extractions

10% shoulder joint

25% elbow

haemarthroses

hepatomegaly due to hepatitis C

5% hip

muscle haematoma

45% knee

haemophilic arthropathy (can affect all joints with previous bleeds)

15% ankle

Figure 9.1 Clinical features of haemophilia.

treatment with the appropriate clotting factor has to be given intra-venously to correct the coagulopathy. Available clotting factors are either recombinant (which are expensive) or plasma derived. Since 1985, plasma-derived products have undergone viral inactivation during their preparation to destroy viruses present in the source plasma. Patients treated prior to 1985 may be infected with hepatitis B or C and HIV infections.

Von Willebrand's disease is an autosomal dominant disorder affecting up to 1% of the population. It is due to a deficiency of von Willebrand factor, a multimeric protein that binds platelets to damaged endothelium. Patients have excessive bruising, nose bleeds, heavy menstrual periods and bleed excessively after trauma, surgery and dental extractions.

Other inherited bleeding disorders are very rare and include deficiencies of any of the other coagulation factors e.g. factor XI, or abnormalities of platelet function such as Glanzmann's thrombasthenia.

Acquired bleeding disorders can be due to thrombocytopenia (e.g. due to autoantibodies in immune thrombocytopenic purpura) or abnormalities of platelet function that are most commonly observed in patients taking aspirin, a drug that irreversibly inhibits the platelet enzyme cyclo-oxygenase; as well as a bleeding tendency, purpura will be seen (see Colour Plate 5). The causes of bleeding in patients with liver disease is multifactorial and complex and include thrombocytopenia, vitamin K deficiency and failure to produce the clotting factors that are normally made in the liver.

Thrombotic disorders

Thrombosis is inappropriate intravascular coagulation. It occurs due to abnormalities in: the vessel wall, the constituents of the blood and blood flow. Arterial thrombosis most commonly results in myocardial infarction (MI) or stroke, while venous thrombosis results in deep vein thrombosis (DVT) of the legs or pulmonary emboli (PE). Disruption of the endothelium is of critical importance in arterial thrombosis while reduced flow and hypercoagulability are more important in venous thrombosis. Risk factors for arterial thrombosis include smoking, obesity, diabetes, hypertension and a high level of cholesterol. Risk factors for venous thrombosis include immobility, surgery, pregnancy, oral contraceptive use and some inherited factors such as Factor V Leiden, the prothrombin

20210A mutation and deficiencies of antithrombin, protein C or protein S.

Anticoagulants

The three most common anticoagulant drugs are aspirin, heparin and warfarin.

Aspirin inhibits platelet function irreversibly through its action on the enzyme cyclo-oxygenase. It causes a prolonged bleeding time and is used in the prevention and treatment of arterial thrombosis.

Heparin is a glycosaminoglycan and acts as an anticoagulant by potentiating the inhibition of thrombin by antithrombin. It can be given intravenously or subcutaneously but not orally. It has an immediate action and is often the first drug used in patients with acute thrombosis. Low molecular weight heparins have recently been introduced which are better absorbed, have less non-specific binding and more predictable pharmacokinetics. They can be given once daily by subcutaneous injection without monitoring even in the presence of acute thrombosis.

Warfarin can only be given orally and acts by inhibiting the synthesis of vitamin K dependent clotting factors (II, VII, IX and X). It has a slow onset of action and a long half-life, so it is given once daily. The daily dose varies widely between individuals. It is monitored with the international normalised ratio (INR) test. The normal INR target for patients with a first thrombosis or atrial fibrillation is 2.0–3.0, while for recurrent thrombosis or mechanical prosthetic heart valves it is 3.0–4.5. The main side effect is bleeding and this can be treated by reducing the INR with vitamin K, fresh frozen plasma or coagulation factor concentrate. It is important to check a patient's INR before performing dental extractions, which can be carried out provided the INR is less than 3.0. Some drugs can interfere with warfarin, for example, erythromycin and metronidazole can enhance the anticoagulant effect of warfarin.

Summary

• **Anaemia** is defined as a low haemoglobin and has many causes; it can produce a smooth tongue or angular stomatitis.
• **Sickle cell disease** is due to an autosomal recessive gene and affects Afro-Caribbeans who get sickle cell crises. Patients need to be well oxygenated during treatment.

- **Leukaemias and lymphomas** are malignant conditions of the white blood cells that can cause gum hypertrophy or tonsillar enlargement.
- **Haemophilia** is a sex-linked bleeding disorder that affects males who get bleeding into joints or muscle or after operations. They can bleed after dental extractions and need factor VIII concentrate. They may be infected with HIV or hepatitis.
- **Von Willebrand's disease** is autosomal dominant, affects 1% of the population and causes excessive bleeding after surgery including dental extraction.
- **Acquired bleeding disorders** can be due to a low platelet count or vitamin K deficiency.
- **Thrombotic disorders** give hypercoaguability, e.g. with venous thrombosis.
- **Anticoagulation** with aspirin will give a prolonged bleeding time and patients receiving heparin will also bleed excessively. Warfarin is given for venous thrombosis, atrial fibrillation and prosthetic heart valves and will cause patients to bleed after surgery. Dental extractions can be done when the INR is less than 3.0.

Further reading

Hoffbrand, A.V., Moss, P., Pettit, J. (2001) *Essential Haematology.* 4th edition. Oxford, Blackwell Science.

Website

Medline bleeding disorders:
http://www.nlm.nih.gov/medlineplus/bleedingdisorders.html

CHAPTER 10
Infectious Diseases

The dentist will often see patients who have a coincidental infection of the face or lips, such as impetigo, or herpes simplex. It is important for the dentist to know the risks of these infections to staff and the patient and what treatment may be appropriate. Other infections that are of particular concern to dentists are hepatitis, HIV, and oral conditions that can result from genitourinary infections.

Facial infections

Impetigo

Impetigo is a pustular infection scattered over the face and legs, usually in children or young adults, due to *Staphylococcus aureus* or *Streptococcus pyogenes* (see Colour Plate 25). The bacteria are usually acquired by direct contact. There can be scanty lesions or widespread crusting. Systemic symptoms are rare. Treatment is with oral co-amoxiclav or ampicillin.

Erysipelas and cellulitis

Erysipelas is severe infection of the superficial skin predominantly due to *Streptococcus pyogenes* but occasionally caused by other streptococci or *S. aureus*. It is mostly seen in children, young adults or the elderly. Its virulence determinants include:
• **protection** from host response by streptokinase, streptolysin and deoxyribonucleases
• **spread** through connective tissues by action of hyaluronidase and proteinase.

Bacteria gain entry through fissures in the skin around the nose or ears. There is an abrupt onset of fever, headache, malaise, sometimes vomiting, with a rapidly enlarging area of redness and swelling on the face, sometimes of both cheeks.

Sometimes the relatively deeper layers of the skin can be affected and the infection can track more widely as a spreading **cellulitis**, particularly when infection involves the neck and chest wall (see Colour Plate 26). If the patient reports that this is a painful process, it is possible that there is a necrotising fasciitis, which is a medical emergency. Treatment of all cases of erysipelas and cellulitis of the head and neck requires requires hospitalisation and intravenous penicillin with flucloxacillin.

Herpes simplex virus (HSV) infection (cold sores)

Cold sores are common and caused by HSV-1 or a closely-related virus, HSV-2, which are transmitted between humans by surface contact to cause a relatively severe 'primary' infection (see Colour Plate 29). In the case of HSV-1, this is usually a pharyngitis or a gingivostomatitis, and is mostly seen in children and young adults. HSV-2 is responsible for most cases of genital herpes and is sexually transmitted, resulting in painful genital ulcers. However, HSV-1 can cause genital infections, and HSV-2 can cause gingivostomatitis.

After the primary infection, the virus persists in the body, i.e. it is **latent**. In the case of HSV-1 it lies dormant in the trigeminal ganglia. Subsequently, the virus is reactivated, traffics along peripheral nerves, and then causes a vesicular eruption at the gingivostomal margin. External stimuli that induce reactivation include:
- bright sunlight and extreme cold
- intercurrent infections, e.g. pneumonia
- stress
- defective cell mediated immunity (e.g. chemotherapy).

Reactivation is sometimes asymptomatic and the virus is shed in the saliva. In herpes labialis (cold sores around the mouth, Figure 10.1) a prodrome of paraesthesiae is followed by painful vesicles which persist for up to a week then heal without scarring. Treatment is with topical aciclovir. For severe primary infection, systemic treatment with oral or intravenous aciclovir may be necessary.

Herpetic whitlow is a painful primary HSV infection of the finger usually seen in healthcare workers such as dentists who have touched a lesion or the mouth of an asymptomatic shedder. It can be severe with systemic features. Herpetic eye infections may be primary or reactivated. Involvement of the cornea is a serious problem. Treatment is with topical aciclovir and an ophthalmologist must be involved.

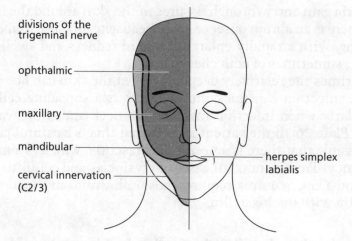

Figure 10.1 Herpes simplex often involves areas around the mouth (right side), while herpes zoster frequently involves one of the divisions of the trigeminal nerve (left side).

Herpes zoster (shingles)

Shingles is caused by a herpes virus (varicella zoster virus: VZV) and is due to reactivation of latent infection (see Colour Plate 30). The virus causes chicken pox mostly in young children and following primary infection, travels along peripheral nerves to lie dormant in dorsal root ganglia. It is estimated that shingles will occur on average once every 40 years. The chances of reactivation are increased by immunosuppression.

The virus reactivates usually in only one dorsal root ganglion. It travels down the related sensory peripheral nerve and causes a severe painful vesicular eruption in the innervated dermatome There is usually a prodrome of pain or paraesthesiae. It never crosses the midline unless the patient has a multidermatome reactivation, as sometimes seen in immunosuppressed patients. The vesicles coalesce, crust and may become secondarily infected.

The commonest sites of reactivation are the thoracic segments and on the face in a division of the trigeminal nerve (Figure 10.1). The vesicles persist for a week and may scar. Extreme pain, post-herpetic neuralgia, can persist for months and years. Sometimes the eye can be involved, requiring ophthalmic assessment. Rarely, facial nerve involvement produces vesicles in the ear, facial nerve palsy, loss of taste over the tongue, and palatal vesicles (Ramsay Hunt syndrome).

Treatment of shingles is with oral famciclovir or ganciclovir, started as soon as possible. Postherpetic neuralgia can be difficult to treat: amitriptyline or opiates may be required.

Fungal infection

The commonest skin fungal infection is tinea pedis (athlete's foot) in which fungi infect the areas between toes and cause fissuring and cracking. Scalp infection, tinea capitis, is common, particularly in children who develop discrete areas of hair loss and scaling. Ringworm is a widespread fungal infection in which there are circular lesions scattered over the body (see Colour Plate 32). Treatment is with a topical antifungal, e.g. miconazole, or, for severe or widespread infection, oral terbinafine or itraconazole.

Facial exanthem

The appearance of the exanthem (rash) is critical. If it is erythematous and spreading, it is usually erysipelas or cellulitis due to streptococci or *Staphylococcus aureus*. If it is composed of multiple small elements that are pustular, the likeliest cause is impetigo (usually *S. aureus* in children); multiple vesicular lesions are usually due to herpes simplex virus. Chicken pox is initially a sparse rash of maculopapular lesions that then evolve into vesicular and finally pustular lesions, with the elements each being in different stages of development.

Chronic skin rashes are usually non-infectious, but can be due to mycobacterial infection or actinomycosis. The latter nowadays is rare, but presents as chronic indurated areas, particularly on the neck, which form sinuses and exude yellowish crusty material (sulphur granules).

Cervical lymphadenopathy

In any patient with cervical lymphadenopathy (see Colour Plate 6), careful inspection of the oral cavity is mandatory, as this may reveal the obvious cause, such as tonsillar swelling or pharyngitis (due to streptococcal pharyngitis or glandular fever due to Epstein–Barr virus, EBV). Occasionally there may be infection of dental spaces that cause lymphadenopathy. Otherwise, lymphadenopathy can be due to systemic diseases. Non-infectious causes include lymphoma or other malignancies. In the case of lymphoma, the nodes are usually rubbery and large.

Systemic infections that cause lymphadenopathy include tuberculosis (TB), EBV, cytomegalovirus (CMV), toxoplasmosis, rubella and *Mycoplasma*. There are many others, but they are generally less common in the UK. In TB, the nodes are usually painless, and may be fluctuant if they contain pus. There may be clinical signs consistent with pulmonary tuberculosis. In EBV, CMV and toxoplasmosis, the nodes are usually slightly tender, and accompanied by general symptoms such as malaise and sore throat. A single very tender node is often due to a deep-seated bacterial infection and should be referred urgently for assessment.

Summary: Facial infections

Impetigo
- pustular and crusted eruption often on face or legs
- mostly due to *Staphylococcus aureus*
- treatment with oral co-amoxiclav

Erysipelas
- skin infection usually due to *Streptococcus pyogenes*
- associated with systemic symptoms, e.g. fever, malaise
- often involves the face or leg
- requires in-patient treatment with intravenous penicillin

Herpes simplex
- 'cold sores' often occur around the mouth
- herpes simplex virus (HSV) 1 may cause pharyngitis or gingivo-stomatitis as primary infection
- HSV 2 generally causes genital infection
- reactivation may be caused by sunlight, stress or reduced immune state
- treatment is with oral (or topical) aciclovir

Herpes zoster
- caused by chickenpox virus that lies dormant in dorsal root ganglia of the spinal cord
- often involves trigeminal nerve distribution
- reactivation may be caused by reduced immune state
- post-herpetic neuralgia is a painful condition that persists after the acute infection has cleared
- treatment is with oral aciclovir

Fungal infection
- dermatophyte fungi cause tinea infection
- different sites involved, e.g. tinea capitis (scalp), tinea pedis (feet), or tinea corporis (body)
- treatment with a topical or systemic antifungal agent

Facial exanthem
- if spreading consider erysipelas or cellulitis
- if vesicular, exclude herpes simplex or chickenpox
- if crusting, it may present as impetigo

Cervical lymphadenopathy
- exclude common infections such as pharyngitis or glandular fever
- examine for lymphoma or other malignancy
- consider other infections such as tuberculosis

Human immunodeficiency virus

Acquired immune deficiency syndrome (AIDS) was first recognised in the USA in 1981 following reports of *Pneumocystis* pneumonia and Kaposi's sarcoma in young homosexual men who had defective cellular immunity. Human immunodeficiency virus (HIV) was identified in 1983 and a diagnostic antibody test developed in 1984. By 1999, over 20,000 people were alive with diagnosed HIV infection in the UK. Anonymous surveys indicate that one third of infections remain undiagnosed. The World Health Organization suggests more than 40 million people are infected worldwide.

The virus

HIV is a retrovirus. Retroviruses are ribonucleic acid (RNA) viruses that code for the enzyme reverse transcriptase, which allows deoxyribonucleic acid (DNA) to be transcribed from RNA. Viral DNA can then be incorporated into the host DNA, so establishing chronic infection. The primary target of HIV is CD4, a cell surface receptor found on T-lymphocytes but also present on monocytes, macrophages, Langerhans cells and dendritic cells, all important in the immune response. HIV binds to CD4 receptors and enters the cell where it uses the reproductive system to manufacture new viral copies, destroying the host cell in the process.

HIV test

The HIV test for antibodies to HIV components becomes positive between three weeks and three months after infection. Testing before three months may not allow sufficient time for antibody production. For all positive results a second specimen is tested to confirm the finding and ensure that the result refers to the correct patient.

Transmission

Globally, heterosexual transmission is the commonest route of HIV acquisition. Transmission can follow:

- percutaneous injury with a contaminated needle
- vertical transmission from mother to baby (usually perinatally)
- receipt of infected blood, organ or semen donations.

Factors that increase the risk of acquisition include the type and frequency of exposure, the HIV stage in the infected individual and the presence of a concurrent sexually transmitted infection. The risk is higher with anal than with vaginal intercourse due to associated trauma, and is greater if the contact has a high viraemia, as seen at seroconversion or in late stages of the disease.

HIV is present in semen, cervical secretions, lymphocytes, cell free plasma, cerebrospinal fluid, tears, saliva, urine and breast milk, but its concentration varies. There is little evidence that HIV is spread by saliva, although cases of HIV acquisition following oro-genital sexual contact are reported. The oral cavity is protected from viral infection by the mucous membranes and antiviral secretions in saliva. However, entry of virus may be increased if there is breach of these defences such as trauma, bleeding or inflammation, e.g. secondary gingivitis, pharyngitis and tonsillitis, mouth ulceration and xerostomia.

Clinical features

Two thirds of people acquiring HIV experience a short illness at the time of seroconversion when antiviral antibodies develop. This may resemble influenza with fever, malaise, arthralgia, lymphadenopathy, macular papular rash, oral or anogenital ulceration or neurological symptoms. Thereafter they may remain asymptomatic for a number of years. The activity of disease can be determined by monitoring the viral load and CD4 cell count. As the disease progresses the CD4 cell count falls and when it drops to levels $<250 \times 10^6/l$ patients become susceptible to opportunistic infections. Table 10.1 shows stages of the disease.

In the UK, AIDS is a clinical diagnosis based on the presence in an HIV-infected individual of an AIDS-defining condition such as: *Pneumocystis carinii* pneumonia, oesophageal candidiasis, Kaposi's sarcoma (see Colour Plate 31), primary cerebral lymphoma, non-Hodgkin's lymphoma, tuberculosis, disseminated myco-bacterial disease, recurrent salmonella septicaemia, HIV wasting syndrome, HIV encephalopathy, recurrent pneumonia within one year, invasive cervical cancer, cytomegalovirus retinitis, cerebral toxoplasmosis, disseminated coccidiomycosis, disseminated histo-plasmosis and isosporiasis with diarrhoea for more than one month.

Table 10.1 The main stages and clinical features of HIV infection

Stage of infection	Clinical features/considerations	Viral load	CD4 count
seroconversion	glandular fever-like illness rash lymphadenopathy arthralgia malaise neurological symptoms	transient moderately raised	good >500
asymptomatic HIV infection	may remain asymptomatic with stable viral load and CD4 count for several years (average 8–10 years)	low	good (>500 but falling)
deterioration in immune function	consideration of antiretroviral medication and prophylactic antibiotics	increasing	decreasing

AIDS	opportunistic infections:
	  oral/oesophageal candidiasis
	  Pneumocystis carinii pneumonia
	  toxoplasmosis
	  cytomegalovirus retinitis
	  tuberculosis
	  disseminated mycobacterial
	    disease
	other AIDS defining illnesses:
	  Kaposi's sarcoma
	  non-Hodgkin's lymphoma
	  cervical cancer
	  HIV wasting syndrome
		high	low

Treatment

The development of highly active anti-retroviral therapy (HAART) and the use of prophylactic therapy to prevent opportunistic infections in patients with low CD4 cell counts has dramatically changed the prognosis for HIV and AIDS. Usual practice is to use a combination of three or more anti-HIV drugs to minimise the development of viral resistance.

Summary: HIV

- **Incidence** of HIV infection is increasing in the UK.
- **Clinical findings** related to the stage of disease and CD4 cell count; opportunistic infections more common if CD4 <250.
- **Transmission** is sexual (vaginal, anal, oral), by needle/blood product/organ donation/inoculation, and vertical.

• **Treatment** with anti-retroviral therapy allows some restoration of immune function, and prophylactic antibiotics reduce opportunistic infections.

• **Prevention** is by encouraging the use of condoms, treating and reducing the incidence of sexually transmitted infection, encouraging the availability of needle exchanges, the screening of blood products for HIV and ensuring a reduction of vertical transmission.

Hepatitis A, B and C

Hepatitis A

Hepatitis A (HAV) is the commonest form of viral hepatitis. Infection is usually asymptomatic or a mild, self-limiting childhood illness with fever, malaise, anorexia, nausea, vomiting and sometimes jaundice or pruritus. Typically liver transaminase enzyme levels are elevated. HAV is not associated with chronic liver disease nor chronic carrier status. The incubation period is 15–50 days. Transmission is by the faeco-oral route. The virus enters the gut and localises in liver hepatocytes where replication occurs. HAV is excreted via the biliary tree to the intestine and is shed in faeces for 1–2 weeks prior to the onset of symptoms and for at least one week afterwards.

Improvements in living conditions have reduced the incidence of childhood HAV. Most adults are not immune to HAV and infection in later life has a higher morbidity and mortality. Vaccination with inactivated virus is recommended for adults travelling to high prevalence areas and in others at risk, e.g. staff in a virus laboratory or individuals with high-risk sexual practices.

Hepatitis B

Hepatitis B virus (HBV) is present in blood and body fluids of infected individuals. Transmission occurs by:
• sexual contact
• percutaneous inoculation with contaminated needles
• transfusion with contaminated blood products
• vertically from mother to baby.

The incubation period is 1–6 months. Symptoms include anorexia, arthralgia, nausea, fever, itching and hepatomegaly.

Mostly the illness is self-limiting, but 5–10% fail to clear the virus and develop chronic hepatitis which can progress to cirrhosis or liver cancer. Serological evidence is required for the diagnosis of HBV infection. Presence of hepatitis B core antibody (HBcAb) indicates previous infection, isolated surface antibody (HbsAb) reveals previous vaccination and persistent surface (HbsAg) or envelope antigen (HbeAg) more than 6 months after infection signifies chronic hepatitis. Preventive vaccination is used in those at risk for HBV, including health care workers, intravenous drug users, those who change sexual partners frequently and close family contacts of HBV carriers.

Hepatitis C

Hepatitis C virus (HCV) is acquired by contact with infected blood, either by needle inoculation, transfusion or via a breach in a skin. Most British cases occur in IV drug users who share equipment. Sexual transmission can occur but is uncommon. Acute infection is frequently unrecognised: there are few associated symptoms. Fifty per cent of people with HCV become chronic carriers. Cirrhosis develops in 20–30% over 5–30 years. Of these, 15% progress to liver cancer. There is no currently available vaccination. Dual therapy with ribavirin and interferon may be given.

Summary: Hepatitis

• **Hepatitis A** is transmitted by the faeco-oral route, there is no chronic carrier state, and no chronic liver damage.
• **Hepatitis B** is transmitted by sexual contact, needle/blood product inoculation or by vertical transmission. Five to ten per cent of those infected become chronic carriers, with a risk of cirrhosis and hepatocellular carcinoma.
• **Hepatitis C** is transmitted by needle/blood product inoculation. Fifty per cent become chronic carriers, 20–30% develop cirrhosis, 15% of whom develop hepatocellular carcinoma.

Oral conditions and genitourinary infection

Oral pathology can occur with sexually transmitted infections such as herpes simplex (see above), gonorrhoea, syphilis, chlamydia and HIV infection. Recognition of signs in the oral cavity alerts the dentist to refer the patient for infection screening and to advise on ways to reduce transmission to partners.

Syphilis

Syphilis is uncommon in the UK. It is usually acquired by sexual contact with an infected person, but can be transmitted vertically from mother to baby. Acquired syphilis begins as a painless ulcer with a raised edge (primary chancre). This is followed by a secondary stage of systemic infection and, several years later, tertiary syphilis develops in 30% of untreated persons, involving either the cardio-vascular or nervous system, or presenting with destructive granu-lomatous lesions know as gummata.

The mouth may be involved at any stage. The primary chancre can occur in the oral cavity following orogenital contact. *Treponema pallidum*, the causative organism, can be identified in serum from the lesion by dark ground microscopy. In secondary syphilis, oral mucous patches described as 'snail track ulcers' can occur on the tongue, tonsils and lips. Mouth lesions of both primary and second-ary syphilis are infectious. In tertiary syphilis, gummata appear as punched-out ulcers that heal with scarring, usually on the hard and soft palate, tongue and uvula.

Gonorrhoea and chlamydia

There is a strong link between orogenital sexual contact and phar-yngeal infection with *Neisseria gonorrhoea*. Gonococcal pharyngitis is usually asymptomatic but 15% of patients have a sore throat and 5% a purulent tonsillitis. Transmission from the throat to the genital area is well described. *Chlamydia trachomatis* infection is the com-monest bacterial sexually transmitted infection in the UK. Most cases are asymptomatic. Pharyngeal infection following receptive oral sex with an infected male partner is well documented.

HIV infection

The oral manifestations of HIV disease vary with the degree of immunosuppression present.

Oral thrush
Colonisation of the oral cavity with *Candida albicans*, the yeast responsible for most cases of thrush is present in 20–50% of healthy individuals. Symptomatic oral candidiasis occurs in immunosup-pressed patients and is common in HIV infection. Broad-spectrum antibiotics and steroids predispose. Several forms of oral candidiasis occur in HIV infection. Pseudomembraneous candidosis is charac-terised by removable white plaques. In hyperplastic candidiasis the white plaques are non-removable. Erythematous candidosis is more difficult to recognise, with smooth depapillated areas on the palate and dorsum of the tongue. An angular cheilitis with cracking and fissuring at the corners of the mouth is common in HIV infec-tion and is usually due to an overgrowth of candida. Oesophageal involvement occurs with more profound immunosuppression.

Oral hairy leucoplakia

Oral hairy leucoplakia (OHL) appears as linear white lesions on the lateral tongue and cannot be removed by abrasion. Up to 40% of HIV patients have some degree of OHL. It is caused by Epstein–Barr virus, is benign and usually asymptomatic. OHL occurs in immuno-suppression due to other conditions and with long-term steroid usage.

Kaposi's sarcoma

Kaposi's sarcoma (KS) is a neoplastic proliferation of endothelial cells triggered by a herpes virus. It occurs in 15% of patients with AIDS. Oral or perioral lesions are often present. Biopsy confirms the diagnosis.

Herpes simplex virus (HSV) infection

In HIV infection, herpes labialis can be severe, frequent and prolonged.

Periodontal disease

Periodontal disease may be an early symptom of HIV infection. The earliest change is linear gingival erythema, followed by necrotising gingivitis and subsequently necrotising periodontitis. Necrotising stomatitis involving adjacent soft tissues and underlying alveolar bone occasionally occurs. There is under-lying anaerobic and aerobic bacterial infection and the condition is progressive, requiring regular dental attention for antibiotics and debridement.

Non-Hodgkin's lymphoma

Non-Hodgkin's lymphoma (NHL) occurs 100 times more frequently in HIV patients than in the general population. Lesions in the oral cavity present as focal soft tissue swellings, which are rapidly progressive.

Mouth ulcers

Recurrent aphthous ulceration may be problematic in HIV-infected individuals and can interfere with speech and swallowing. Other causes include infection with herpes simplex virus, varicella zoster and cytomegalovirus. Drugs may induce iatrogenic oral ulceration. Syphilis should be excluded.

Summary: Sexually transmitted infections

• **Mouth and pharynx** may show clinical signs of sexually transmitted infections (STIs) and act as a route of transmission.

• **Oral problems associated with HIV infection** include: oral candidiasis, angular cheilitis, oral hairy leucoplakia, Kaposi's sarcoma, herpes simplex infection, periodontal disease, non-Hodgkin's lymphoma and mouth ulcers.

• **Health education** on reduction of transmission of STIs is important for patients with oral lesions.

Further reading

Adler, M.W. (1997) *ABC of Sexually Transmitted Diseases.* 3ʳᵈ edition. London, BMJ Publishing.

Alder, M.W. (ed) (1997) *ABC of AIDS.* 4ᵗʰ edition. London, BMJ Publishing.

Edwards, S., Carne, C. (1998) Oral sex and the transmission of viral (and non-viral) STIs. *Sex Transm Inf* 74, 6–10 and 95–100.

Greenspan, D., Greenspan, J.S. (1996) HIV-related oral disease. *Lancet,* 348, 729–33.

Harahap, M. (ed) (1997) *Diagnosis and Treatment of Skin Infections.* Oxford, Blackwell Science, 1997.

Ryder, S.D., Beckingham, I.J. (2001) Chronic viral hepatitis. *Br Med J* 322, 219–21.

Websites

Aidsmap: http://www.aidsmap.com
Erysipelas: http://www.emedicine.com/derm/topic129.htm
Health Protection Agency: http://www.phls.co.uk/
Hepatitis:
   http://dir.yahoo.com/Health/Diseases_and_Conditions/Hepatitis/
Herpes simplex:
   http://www.dermnet.org.nz/dna.herpes.simplex/hsimpl.html

CHAPTER 11
Allergy

Dentists often encounter allergic problems, so the ability to recognise allergic reactions and to limit their occurrence is important for all dentists.

Types of hypersensitivity reaction

Type I hypersensitivity (immediate or IgE-mediated) is due to the release of vasoactive substances (typically histamine) by mast cells after antigen-specific immunoglobulin E (IgE) molecules on the cell surface are cross-linked by the antigen in question (Figure 11.1) Urticaria is the usual result but angioedema and even life-threatening anaphylactic shock can result.

Type II hypersensitivity (antibody-dependent cytotoxicity) is responsible for blistering conditions such as pemphigus in which oral blistering and subsequent ulceration are common.

Type III hypersensitivity is mediated by circulating immune complexes comprised of antigen and antibody. It is a mechanism for vasculitis that can present in the mouth.

Type IV hypersensitivity (cell-mediated or delayed type) is due to specifically-sensitised T-lymphocytes, e.g. as in allergic contact dermatitis to a topical preparation applied to facial skin, or oral lichenoid reaction to mercury in amalgam.

Drug reactions may be due to one of more of the above hypersensitivity mechanisms. They will not be dealt with in this chapter.

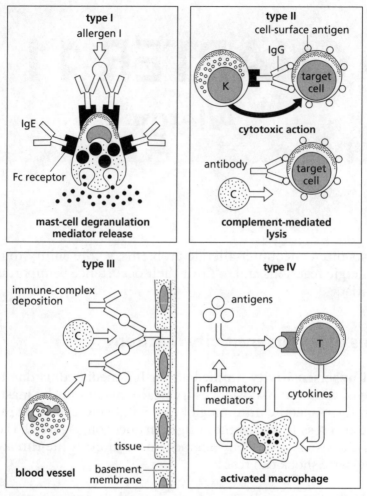

Figure 11.1 The four types of hypersensitivity reaction.

Symptoms and signs

At the initial consultation, all patients should be asked if they have
a history of any allergic reactions, for example to oral medicaments
(e.g. a drug eruption as shown in Colour Plate 35), topical agents
including cosmetics and to rubber (e.g. in rubber gloves). It is also
useful to ask about atopic tendency, i.e. a history of childhood
eczema, asthma or hay fever and/or a family history of allergies. For
the dental profession, the most frequently-encountered types of
allergic reaction will be immediate and cell-mediated.

Immediate-type hypersensitivity

Type I (immediate) hypersensitivity (Figure 11.1) is an acute phenomenon and can be manifested as acute swelling and erythema of

the skin or angioedema (more prominent swelling, e.g. of the lips or throat as shown in Colour Plate 33) if the allergy is severe. These signs can come on within 5–20 minutes of contact with the offending allergen and may be accompanied by signs of shock, such as weak pulse, falling blood pressure, clamminess, feeling faint and sick. The patient may collapse and go into shock and there can be difficulty in breathing due to swelling of the upper airway and throat. These are the signs of an acute anaphylactic reaction.

Examples in dental practice are **allergy to latex** and some **food allergies** (e.g. to peanut). Latex allergy can be serious and even life-threatening and so it is essential that the dentist can recognise when these complications may occur and how they should be managed. Immediate hypersensitivity to local anaesthetics is very uncommon.

Cell-mediated hypersensitivity

A typical example of type IV (cell-mediated) hypersensitivity is **allergic contact dermatitis**. The signs of a contact dermatitis can come on over a period of hours or days and would be manifest on the face as redness with scaling and some swelling of the skin, possibly with the presence of small blisters (i.e. the changes of an eczema, as shown in Colour Plate 41).

If a contact dermatitis is more chronic, then the acute changes of redness and swelling are replaced by thickening of the skin with more prominent scaling. These changes can affect the lips, cheeks, eyelids, ears or any other part of the anatomy. Examples in dental practice include allergy to metal (e.g. nickel or palladium) used in orthodontic materials and occasionally allergy to dental plastics used in dentures.

In intraoral lichenoid reactions ('lichen planus'), the changes are of a white papular eruption on the buccal or gingival mucosa (see Colour Plate 45). A clue that this might be a type IV cell-mediated response could be a lichenoid change present on the buccal or gingival mucosa and adjacent to an amalgam restoration. Mercury in amalgam and gold in capped teeth are causes of this lichenoid type of cell-mediated reaction.

Summary: Allergy

• **Type I (immediate, IgE-mediated) hypersensitivity** is characterised by histamine release from mast cells. It produces urticaria, angioedema or, if severe, anaphylaxis. Dental examples are latex allergy and food allergy.

• **Type II (antibody-dependent cytotoxicity) hypersensitivity** is mediated by antibodies to target cells that induce cell or complement-mediated damage. A dental example is pemphigus.

• **Type III (immune complex disease) hypersensitivity:** The combination of antigens and antibodies in the blood (immune complexes) lodge in small vessels causing damage. In dental practice this may be seen as vasculitis in the mouth.

• **Type IV (cell-mediated, delayed) hypersensitivity:** Sensitised T cells have contact with an antigen via antigen-presenting cells and produce inflammation. Dental examples are an oral contact dermatitis to nickel in orthodontic wire and lichenoid reaction to mercury in amalgam.

Further reading

Shah, M., Lewis, F.M., Gawkrodger, D.J. (1996) Contact allergy in patients with oral symptoms. *Am J Cont Dermatitis* 7, 146–51.

Website

Latex allergy links: http://latexallergylinks.tripod.com/
Oral lichen planus:
  http://www.medicine.org.hk/hksdv/bulletins/200212-05.pdf

CHAPTER 12
Ophthalmological Diseases

Patients may present incidentally to the dentist with an eye problem that requires urgent referral. The ability to make a brief assessment of eye disease is helpful to the dentist.

Ophthalmic history

As in all areas of medicine a careful history is important. In particular one needs to ask specifically for visual disturbance – 'When was the vision in that eye good?' This will differentiate a long-standing defect from a new symptom. The following points in the history are important (Table 12.1):

- **floaters** – sudden onset suggests posterior vitreous detachment with a risk of retinal detachment. Consider vitreous haemorrhage if associated with loss of vision
- **flashing lights** – transient, associated with head or eye movements, suggests vitreous detachment; recurrent for several minutes often in zig-zag or vivid patterns is usually migraine
- **loss of visual field** – indicates serious pathology; note whether loss of vision is acute or gradual
- **pain** – suggests serious pathology such as corneal ulceration, iritis, or acute glaucoma. It is important to differentiate pain from discomfort or a 'gritty' feeling
- **discharge** – clear or purulent, unilateral or bilateral
- **injury** – any history of trauma, how the injury was sustained. If injury sustained while using a hammer or chisel, always suspect high velocity particle causing penetrating injury. With a forceful blunt injury, e.g. a punch, suspect 'blow out fracture'
- **ocular history** – note contact lens wear, high myopia, eye drops and operations

Table 12.1 Common presentations of eye problems or signs

Findings	Interpretation
reduced visual acuity	
improves with pinhole test	refractive cause, new spectacles needed

doesn't improve with pinhole test	suggests pathology:
	  poor red reflex with gradual loss is
	    usually cataract

red eye	
entire conjunctiva – globe and lid	conjunctivitis, subconjunctival haemorrhage from trauma
confined to a sector of the globe	episcleritis, scleritis, subconjunctival haemorrhage
confined to area around limbus ('circumcorneal congestion')	iritis, acute glaucoma
fluorescein staining of cornea	abrasion/ulceration infiltrate suggests infection
irregular pupil	iritis, prior surgery trauma

relative afferent pupillary
  defect present
	optic nerve lesion or large retinal
	  detachment

diminished red reflex	cataract corneal opacity obscures iris and pupil vitreous opacity may indicate haemorrhage

Ophthalmic examination

Ideally special equipment is required, such as Snellen eye chart to record visual acuity, a bright torch, a magnifying aid, e.g. loupe or a direct ophthalmoscope with the +10 lens, cotton buds or paper clip to help lid eversion and fluorescein-impregnated strips or eye drops. These are not likely to be available in the dental practice and so basic methods may need to suffice.

The examination ideally consists of an assessment of vision that includes:
• using Snellen's chart (vision of 6/6 does not exclude serious pathology, even perforating injuries: the pinhole test gives an idea of the potential vision)
• a check on the pupillary reactions
• eversion of the upper eye lid to look for a 'subtarsal' foreign body
• an examination of the cornea, the red reflex and fundus if possible.

Patients who have suffered facial trauma require:
- an assessment of the pupillary reflexes including examination for a relative afferent pupillary defect (RAPD). Constriction of the pupil on the stimulated side is the direct light reflex, constriction of the other pupil is the consensual light reflex
- an inspection of ocular movements
- a check for diplopia
- delineation of the visual fields by confrontation.

Red eye

The patient presenting with a red eye is a common scenario (see Colour Plate 39). The main causes and features are set out in Table 12.2 and Figure 12.1. For dentists in hospital maxillofacial practice, subconjunctival haemorrhage as a result of a fractured zygoma is likely to be the commonest cause of a red eye. Such patients often also have diplopia.

Visual loss or disturbance

It is important to differentiate acute from gradual loss of vision (Figure 12.2). In gradual loss of vision an uncorrected refractive error may be the cause. This is not associated with any other symptoms, and acuity improves with a pinhole. Macular disease and some forms of cataract affect near vision more than distance. Complaints of glare, vision worse in bright light and distance vision affected more than near vision all suggest cataract. The common form of glaucoma does not reduce visual acuity unless it is advanced. It is usually picked up by opticians because of a raised intraocular pressure (IOP), abnormal optic discs or abnormal visual fields.
- **Sudden** loss of vision suggests arterial vascular occlusion.
- **Recurrent transient loss** suggests embolism or ischaemic optic neuropathy.
- **Vein occlusions** are less dramatic in onset, and often present as a symptom with uncertain onset that has been suddenly noticed.
- **Profound loss** suggests arterial occlusion, vitreous haemorrhage or retinal detachment. Other causes usually cause blurring.
- **Distorted vision** suggests macular disease.
- **Loss of left or right field** suggests a hemianopia, often due to a cerebrovascular cause.
- **Progressive loss** starting in the periphery and extending centrally is caused by retinal detachment.
- **Acute glaucoma** is associated with a painful red eye, and nausea.
- **Giant cell arteritis** presents headache, jaw claudication and transient to permanent visual loss in an older patient.

Table 12.2 Causes and features of red eye

Diagnosis	Pattern of redness	Other features	Symptoms	Treatment
conjunctivitis	diffuse including tarsal plate	bilateral, cold symptoms, discharge	burning, gritty, foreign body sensation	topical antibiotics usually
episcleritis	sectoral pinkness	± nodules, no discharge	aching, bruising	oral NSAIDs or referral for topical steroids
scleritis	sectoral deep purple	± nodules ± scleral thinning, no discharge	severe pain	oral steroids/NSAIDs
keratitis	circumcorneal	corneal epithelial defect or infiltrate or foreign body, discharge if infected	photophobia, foreign body sensation	urgent referral if infected, abrasions heal spontaneously or with topical antibiotics
anterior uveitis	circumcorneal	miosed pupil, keratic precipitates, flare, cells, no discharge	photophobia, aching	referral for topical steroids + mydriatics
acute glaucoma	diffuse	fixed mid-dilated pupil, corneal oedema, no discharge	severe pain, nausea, haloes	urgent referral for pupil constriction, reduction of intraocular pressure and laser iridotomy

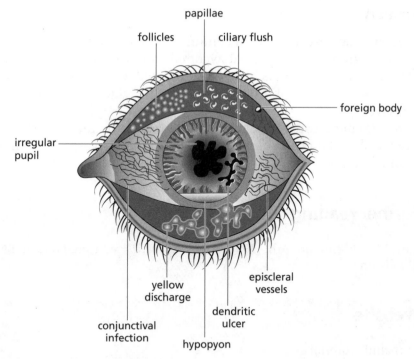

Figure 12.1 Signs of red eye.

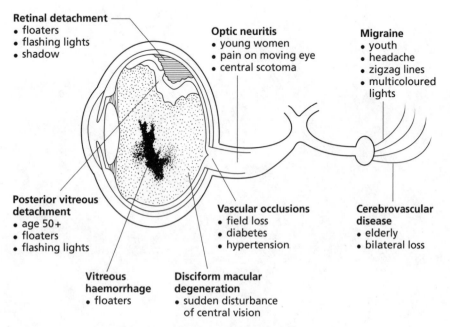

Figure 12.2 Causes of acute visual disturbance.

Summary

- **Red eye** can result from subconjunctival haemorrhage secondary to facial trauma (e.g. fractured zygoma), conjunctivitis (may give a gritty feeling), episcleritis (may be associated with an ache or bruising), iritis (produces photophobia), or acute glaucoma (associated with severe pain).
- **Irregular pupil** can be due to iritis, trauma or previous surgery.
- **Reduced visual acuity** can be caused by a refractive error, cataract or retinal disease.

Further reading

Khaw, P.T., Elkington, A.R. (1997) *ABC of Eyes*. 2nd edition. London, BMJ Publishing.

Website

Ophthalmic tutorials:
http://www.lei.org.au/~leiiweb/teaching/undergrad/index.htm

CHAPTER 13
Ear, Nose and Throat Diseases

The nose warms, humidifies and cleans inspired air, and is the organ of smell. The ear is the organ of hearing and balance. The nose and ears are closely associated with the mandible and their diseases are of relevance to dentists.

Anatomy

The nose consists of the external nose and the paired nasal cavities. The nasal septum divides the nasal cavity into two halves. The roof of the nasal cavities is formed by the nasal cartilages, nasal and frontal bones, cribiform plate of the ethmoid and the body of the sphenoid. The floor is formed by the roof of the oral cavity.

The lateral wall of the nose has three bony projections (turbinates) which serve to increase the surface area of the nasal mucosa. The paranasal sinuses are paired and comprise the frontal, maxillary, ethmoidal and sphenoidal sinuses. (Figure 13.1). The sense of smell is mediated via the olfactory nerve. Somatosensory innervation is via the trigeminal nerve and secretory via the sympathetic and parasympathetic systems.

The ear is divided anatomically into three parts, the external, middle and inner ear. (Figure 13.2). The tympanic membrane (eardrum) divides the external from the middle ear. The inner ear contains the cochlea (organ of hearing) and the vestibular system (the organ of balance) and their central connections. These organs are embedded in dense bone.

Signs and symptoms

The major nasal symptoms include obstruction, discharge (rhinor-rhoea), alterations in the sense of smell, bleeding (epistaxis), facial

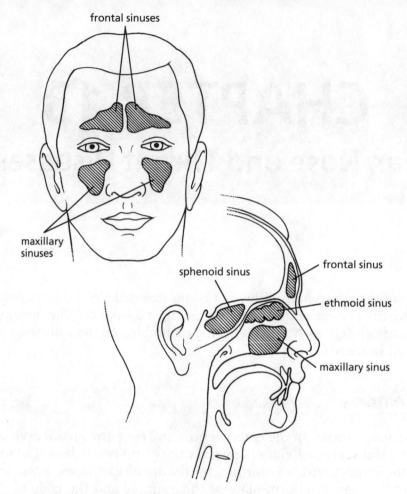

Figure 13.1 The paranasal sinuses.

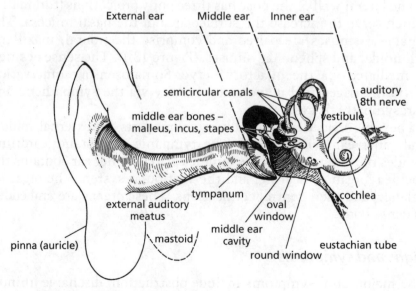

Figure 13.2 Structure of the ear.

pain and cosmetic deformity of the nose. When examining the nose, note the overall shape and the patency of the nasal cavities, the state of the nasal septum and lateral wall of the nose, the nasal mucosa and the presence of secretions or nasal polyps. Patients may complain of hearing loss, otalgia (pain), otorrhoea (discharge), vertigo (dizziness) and tinnitus. Hearing is assessed using tuning forks but details are not discussed here.

Common disorders

Rhinosinusitis

The nasal cavities and paranasal sinuses function as one unit and pathological changes within the nose often also affect the sinus mucosa, hence the term rhinosinusitis. Most cases of sinusitis are due to pathology within the nasal cavities, particularly of the osteomeatal complex, which will lead to alteration in the ventilation and drainage of the large dependent paranasal sinuses.

When this affects the maxillary sinus the patient often complains of a dull throbbing pain in the infraorbital region. This can also be associated with discomfort in the upper dentition which is closely related to the maxillary sinus. Treatment is with decongestants, analgesia and antibiotics when required.

Allergic rhinitis

This is an immunoglobulin E (IgE) mediated hypersensitivity reaction which leads to degranulation of mast cells and the release of vasoactive substances. Allergic rhinosinusitis can either be seasonal – such as hayfever – or perennial – all year round. It is commonly caused by house dustmite or pet fur from cats and dogs. The treatment of allergic rhinitis is allergen avoidance if practical, topical intranasal steroids and antihistamines.

Vasomotor and infective rhinitis

Vasomotor rhinitis is due to an imbalance in the autonomic nervous supply to the nose, leading to nasal obstruction and thickened secretions. Treatment is with intranasal steroids. Infective rhinitis can be due to viral (e.g. common cold), bacterial or fungal infection. Viral and bacterial rhinitis are usually self limiting and resolve spontaneously. Fungal and occasionally bacterial rhinitis will require the appropriate antibiotic and antifungal treatment.

Sinusitis

When inflammatory changes spread from the nasal mucosa to the larger sinuses, sinusitis occurs. Patients may complain of facial pain and this may present to the dentist. In the acute stage there may be tenderness on palpation over the maxillary or frontal sinuses. In chronic sinusitis, a purulent discharge from the front and back of the nose is accompanied by nasal obstruction and sometimes headaches or facial discomfort.

Treatment is with topical nasal decongestants and humidification to remove secretions and improve ventilation, and broad spectrum antibiotics for infection. Surgical drainage of the sinuses is occasionally required.

Nasal trauma

Following trauma it is important to ascertain whether this is localised to the nose or part of more significant facial, neck and body trauma. Patients usually complain of cosmetic deformity, nasal swelling, nasal obstruction, pain and bleeding. Dental trauma may co-exist. Most cases of nasal deformity can be manipulated back into a reasonable position either under local or general anaesthetic.

Epistaxis (nose bleed)

This can be due to either local or general causes. Local causes are usually due to trauma, either infective, digital, nasal fractures or postsurgical. General causes include anticoagulation or haematological disease.

Deafness

This can be one of:
- **conductive** hearing loss – caused by failure of transmission of the sound energy from the outside world to the inner ear and will be due to a variety of causes.
- **sensorineural** hearing loss – due to degeneration of tiny hair cells within the cochlea and their central connections, as happens in the ageing process.
- **mixed** hearing loss – a mixture of the two at the same time.

Vertigo and tinnitus

This describes the hallucination of movement either of the environment around the patient or the patient within the environment and is a symptom of peripheral vestibular disease. Tinnitus is the symptom of noises within the ears or head and is commonly associated with some degeneration of cochlear function.

Impacted wax or foreign body in the external ear

This is often caused by cleaning the ear with cotton buds and can result in conductive hearing loss, pain and discomfort. Wax can usually be softened with olive oil, sodium bicarbonate ear drops, or proprietary cerumolytics and removed by syringing if necessary.

A foreign body in the external ear is more common in children, who may insert foreign bodies into the ears at play and require instrumental removal.

Infection and trauma to the external ear

Infection of the external auditory canal is termed otitis externa and if localised may be due to *Staphylococcus aureus* infection. Generalised otitis externa can either be part of a general skin condition such as psoriasis, a contact dermatitis, or be related to local infection within the ear canal which can either be bacterial, viral or fungal.

Otitis media

Acute otitis media is due to an acute infection of the middle ear cleft – either viral or bacterial – and results in marked otalgia and a conductive hearing loss. The condition may either resolve, with the pain subsiding and the bulging eardrum returning to normal, or progress to tympanic membrane rupture and otorrhoea.

Chronic otitis media, otitis media with effusion (glue ear), is common in childhood and is usually relatively asymptomatic apart from a conductive hearing loss. Most cases resolve spontaneously.

Middle ear effusions in adults

These commonly follow upper respiratory tract infections and resolve spontaneously

Chronic suppurative otitis media is divided into safe and unsafe. If unsafe, it must be managed in an ENT clinic. It is associated with cholesteatoma and destructive processes in and beyond the middle ear cleft. The safe variety is due to a tympanic membrane perforation and there is intermittent discharge due to infection of the mucosa in the middle ear space.

Maxillary sinus carcinoma

Cancer of the nasal cavities and paranasal sinuses is rare and constitutes approximately 3% of head and neck tumours. The majority of tumours (80%) are squamous cell carcinoma, most arising from the maxillary antrum. The presentation of sinonasal malignancy would depend upon the site at which the tumour is found. If found within the nasal cavities, tumours often present with nasal symptoms such as obstruction and epistaxis.

Dentists may occasionally see tumours arising in the maxillary antrum, particularly if there is spread to involve the palate and alveolus. This may result in either an ill-fitting denture or loose teeth. If the tumour extends anteriorly there may be blockage of the nasolacrimal apparatus with epiphora, although facial swelling and distorted sensation of the infraorbital nerve distribution are more likely. Posterior spread into the temporal fossa and skull base can lead to involvement of the pterygoid muscles and trismus. The management of sinonasal disease is best concentrated into head and neck units with specialist knowledge and experience in the management of these tumours.

Summary: Ear nose and throat diseases

• **Anatomy**: the nose consists of the external nose and the paired nasal cavities. The ear is divided into the external, middle and inner ear.
• **Symptoms** of ear and nose problems include nasal obstruction and discharge, altered sense of smell, nose bleed, facial pain, nasal deformity, deafness, vertigo and tinnitus.
• **Allergic rhinitis** is an allergen-specific IgE-mediated hypersensitivity reaction in which sneezing or nasal obstruction occur, e.g. due to housedust mite allergy.
• **Vasomotor rhinitis** is due to an imbalance in the autonomic nervous system leading to nasal obstruction and secretion. Infection can result in similar symptoms to allergic rhinitis.
• **Nasal trauma** may give deformity, swelling, obstruction, pain and bleeding. Dental trauma may co-exist. Most nasal fractures can be manipulated back under anaesthetic.
• **Nosebleed** may be due to local causes, e.g. trauma or infection, or general causes, e.g. bleeding disorder or anticoagulants.

- **Deafness** may be conductive – failure of transmission of the sound – or sensorineural – loss of the tiny hair cells in the cochlea or nerve damage, or both.
- **Otitis media** is an infection of the middle ear, characterised by ear pain and sometimes rupture of the tympanic membrane. It can become chronic and be a cause of conductive deafness.
- **Middle ear effusion** may be associated with infection. The 'unsafe' variety can be associated with the formation of cholesteatoma.
- **Maxillary sinus carcinoma** may present with nasal symptoms (blockage, bleeding, discharge), palatal swelling or loosening of teeth.

Reference

Dhillon, R.S., East, C.A. (1994) *Ear, Nose and Throat and Head and Neck Surgery: an Illustrated Colour Text*. Edinburgh, Churchill Livingstone.

Website

Medline: http://www.nlm.nih.gov/medlineplus/earnoseandthroat.html

CHAPTER 14
Dermatological Diseases

Dentists will be familiar with several common skin diseases as they look at the faces of their patients. They will also need to know about some important conditions that affect both the skin and the oral mucosa.

Facial eruptions

Acne and rosacea

Acne vulgaris is characterised by papules, pustules, comedones, cysts and scars over the cheeks, forehead and chin (Figure 14.1, see also Colour Plate 44). Rosacea, a similar but unrelated condition in which the symptom of facial burning is common, shows erythema, telangiectasia, papules and pustules, especially on the forehead, nose and chin.

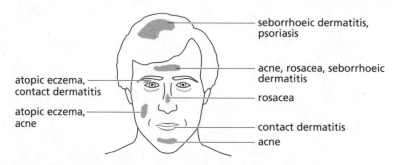

Figure 14.1 The sites of common eruptions on the face.

Eczemas

Atopic eczema, the commonest type of eczema, is characterised by dryness and redness of the skin. Patients complain of a lot of itching, which can lead to thickening of the skin with accentuated crease marks and lichenification, especially on eyelids. In seborrhoeic dermatitis, there is a scaly itchy rash on the scalp, face and presternal areas. Allergic contact dermatitis can give a facial eruption, e.g. due to perfume or cosmetic allergy.

Infections

Facial infections are common. They include bacterial, e.g. impetigo, a superficial infection by *Staphylococcus aureus*, in which yellow crusts form, erysipelas, a form of cellulitis usually due to a beta-haemolytic streptococcus, and boils and folliculitis usually caused by a staphylococcal infection of hair follicles. Viral infections are also common, e.g. cold sores (herpes simplex), and shingles (herpes zoster).

Connective tissue diseases

Systemic lupus erythematosus (SLE) produces the typical 'butterfly' rash on the cheeks (see Colour Plate 11). The condition can affect internal organs including the joints, kidneys, nervous system, lungs and the blood. In discoid lupus erythematosus, a related disorder, there are round scaly raised patches on light-exposed areas. Systemic sclerosis (scleroderma) can affect the face, showing a tight shiny appearance to the skin, with a beaked nose, purse-string mouth and telangiectasia. In dermatomyositis, an inflammatory disease of the skin and muscles, purple discoloration of the eyelids is seen, sometimes with swelling. In patients over 40 years of age with this condition, 40% have an underlying cancer.

Other inflammatory skin diseases

Psoriasis frequently affects the scalp and occasionally the face. Well-defined reddish or purple plaques with silvery scale are seen (see Colour Plate 43). Drug eruptions can affect the face, particularly when they are caused by photosensitivity (e.g. due to thiazide diuretics, non-steroidal anti-inflammatory agents or ACE inhibitors).

Lip disease

Angioedema may cause the lips to swell, sometimes with swelling of the eyelids (see Colour Plate 33). In extreme cases there may be oedema of the larynx and pharynx. If this occurs, emergency measures may be needed, e.g. intramuscular adrenaline. The cause of angioedema is often not found but it is sometimes due to food allergies or allergy to latex.

In granulomatous cheilitis there is swelling of the entire lip. This condition is sometimes associated with Crohn's disease. Dermatitis of the lip may be caused by a contact dermatitis e.g. to a constituent of lipstick. Sometimes there are benign pigmented macules on the lips or small venous 'lakes' characteristically seen to one side of the lower lip.

Tumours of the face and lips

Benign pigmented (melanocytic) naevi are common on the face. Vascular naevi such as strawberry naevus (cavernous haemangioma), the port wine stain, (capillary haemangioma) and spider naevus (see Colour Plate 13) are well known. Viral warts may occur on the face or lips, as can pyogenic granulomas, which actually consist of inflammatory masses of immature capillaries that may follow minor trauma. Seborrhoeic warts are common benign brown warty lesions often seen on the faces of old people. Malignant tumours frequently occur on the face, the commonest being basal cell carcinoma ('rodent ulcer', see Colour Plate 48).

Squamous cell carcinomas are much less common but can grow rapidly and metastasise. Lentigo maligna is a premalignant stage of malignant melanoma on the head and neck. Malignant melanoma (see Colour Plate 47) on the face usually develops from a lentigo maligna in elderly person.

Dermatoses affecting the skin and oral mucosa

Primary bullous disorders

Immunologically-mediated blistering diseases, most importantly bullous pemphigoid, pemphigus and dermatitis herpetiformis, may all involve the oral mucosa with blistering or ulceration. Oral involvement is most frequent in pemphigus, occurring in about 90% of cases. In the commonest type of pemphigoid, there is blistering in about 10%, although there is a rare disorder, cicatricial pemphigoid, in which the conjunctivae, mouth and sometimes other sites are often involved by blistering and scarring (see Colour Plate 40).

In dermatitis herpetiformis, a blistering disorder associated with coeliac disease and gluten sensitive enteropathy, aphthous ulceration is a feature but patients usually have a widespread rash and intractable pruritus. Bullous pemphigoid is commonest in elderly people. Characterised by large tense blisters frequently associated with widespread erythema and pruritus, it is caused by circulating antibodies to skin basement membrane proteins. Pemphigus has a wider age range, is associated with small flaccid blisters and circulating antibodies to skin desmosomes.

Connective tissue disorders

The mouth may be involved in lupus erythematosus (LE) of all types (see Colour Plate 11). In cutaneous forms of LE (e.g. chronic discoid LE), oral mucosal lesions are found in 50% or more of cases. In systemic sclerosis (generalised scleroderma), patients may complain of difficulty in opening the mouth and often suffer from a dry mouth (sicca syndrome).

Lichenoid eruptions

Most but not all patients with cutaneous lichen planus have oral lesions. Oral lichen planus without skin involvement is common (see Colour Plate 45). Lichen planus and atypical lichenoid reactions may be induced by drugs although the commonest (classic) form is of unknown cause. Allergy to mercury in amalgam and to gold can cause lichenoid reactions of the buccal mucosa, tongue, lip or gum adjacent to the restoration or capped tooth.

Infections

Herpes zoster of the trigeminal distribution may be accompanied by an eruption on the palate. Herpes simplex (see Colour Plate 29) may involve the lips or the mouth, causing a gingivitis. Ulcers on the palate are a feature of syphilis. HIV infection is associated with several types of oral lesion including hairy leukoplakia, oral candidiasis and Kaposi's sarcoma (see Colour Plate 31).

Other conditions

Drug reactions, as well as involving the skin, may affect the mouth, especially fixed drug eruptions in which blistering around or inside the mouth can be a feature. Various forms of epidermolysis bullosa can cause blistering of the buccal mucosa (and also the oesophagus). Vasculitis, a generalised disorder caused by damage to blood vessels from circulating immune complex deposition (see Colour Plate 12), may affect the oral mucosa as may erythema multiforme (known as the Stevens–Johnson syndrome when there is prominent oral involvement), which is shown in Colour Plate 36. Blisters and erosions of the oral and other mucosal surfaces are an important component in the rare and serious condition of toxic epidermal necrolysis. Scurvy can cause bleeding gums as well as other signs (see Colour Plate 18).

Swelling of the mouth and lips

Angioedema, often associated with urticaria (nettle rash, hives), frequently affects the tongue, mouth or lips, producing acute swellings that may take several hours to subside. Angioedema may be due to a food allergy (e.g. type I hypersensitivity to peanuts or latex), a drug reaction (e.g. aspirin), or an inherited deficiency of complement components (hereditary angioedema), but often no specific cause is found. Chronic swellings of the lips may occur with eczema, allergic contact dermatitis or granulomatous cheilitis. Patients with lip eczema may have a personal or family history of atopy (hay fever, asthma or eczema). Patch-testing may be required to determine whether there is an allergic contact dermatitis (type IV hypersensitivity).

Pigmentation of the mouth and lips

Pigmentation of the buccal mucosa is normal in individuals with darker skin types. Buccal pigmentation is also noted in Addison's disease and in Peutz–Jeghers syndrome. In the latter condition, macular pigmentation of the lips and buccal mucosa (and sometimes on the fingers) is associated with intestinal polyps which may cause intussusception or be premalignant. Occasionally, drug-induced pigmentation may affect the buccal mucosa (e.g. minocycline).

Summary: Dermatological diseases

- Common **facial eruptions** include acne, eczema, impetigo, boils, and herpes simplex.
- Rare but important **facial rashes** include lupus erythematosus, systemic sclerosis and dermatomyositis.
- Common **facial tumours** include melanocytic naevi, viral warts, seborrhoeic warts, portwine stain naevi and basal cell carcinomas.
- A rarer but important facial tumour is **lentigo maligna**, which can progress to invasive malignant melanoma.
- **Primary blistering eruptions** that affect skin and oral mucosa include pemphigus vulgaris (90% have oral lesions), bullous pemphigoid (10% have oral blisters), cicatricial pemphigoid (all have

mucosal bullae) and dermatitis herpetiformis (aphthous ulcers common).

• **Connective tissue disorders** such as lupus erythematosus often affect both skin and oral mucosa. Patients with systemic sclerosis frequently have a dry mouth.

• **Oral lichenoid reactions** can be due to allergy to mercury in amalgam or to gold.

• **Lip eruptions** include angioedema (e.g. due to food allergy), granulomatous cheilitis (associated with Crohn's disease) and contact dermatitis (e.g. due to a component of lipstick).

Reference

Gawkrodger, D.J. (2002) Dermatology: An Illustrated Colour Text. 3rd edition. Edinburgh, Churchill Livingstone.

Website

Pemphigus:
http://www.usc.edu/hsc/dental/opath/Cards/PemphigusVulgaris.html

CHAPTER 15
Rheumatological Diseases

Rheumatological conditions often have an effect on the mouth through a number of different mechanisms, and the care of patients with rheumatic disorders may present a challenge to dentists. There may be problems from the joints themselves or from mucosal lesions associated with the rheumatic disease.

Rheumatoid arthritis

Rheumatoid arthritis (RA), the commonest inflammatory arthritis, affects 1% of adults in the UK, with a female:male ratio of 3:1. The cause is unknown but there is evidence of genetic predisposition with an association with human leucocyte antigen HLA-DR4. Chronic inflammation in the synovium (the lining of the joint) invades the adjacent articular cartilage and bone, resulting in erosions. The inflammatory process is mediated by cytokines, e.g. tumour necrosis factor (TNF) alpha and interleukin-1.

Clinical features

Rheumatoid arthritis is a systemic disease but joint involvement dominates. It commonly presents with a symmetrical inflammatory arthritis of the small joints of the hands and feet which later spreads to involve large joints. All synovial joints can be affected (Figure 15.1). The disease follows a chronic and variable course. Untreated, persistent joint inflammation damages the articular cartilage, bone and soft tissue, resulting in permanent joint deformity, pain and disability.

Patients complain of joint pain, swelling, morning stiffness and disability. The temporomandibular joints (TMJs) are affected in 25% of cases, usually bilaterally, and cause pain on chewing with no

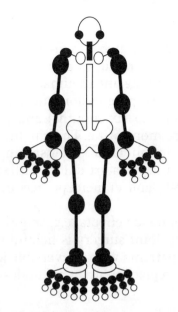

Figure 15.1 Joint involvement.

significant disability. Rarely, joint damage can lead to malalignment of teeth with malocclusion. In juvenile chronic arthritis, there may be underdevelopment of the jaw leading to micrognathism.

Cervical spine involvement can result in subluxation, usually at the atlanto-axial level, and can lead to spinal cord compression. Extra care should be taken in handling the neck in patients with advanced RA, especially during procedures which involve neck extension, e.g. induction of anaesthesia. X-rays of the cervical spine should be taken in flexion and extension pre-operatively to detect increased anterioposterior movement of the odontoid peg and for segmental subluxation. Extra-articular features include secondary Sjogren's syndrome manifested by ocular and oral dryness, rheumatoid nodules, scleritis, fibrosing alveolitis and systemic vasculitis.

Diagnosis

The diagnosis is made clinically on the basis of symmetrical polyarthritis lasting more than six weeks. Rheumatoid factor is detected in the sera of 80% of patients. Patients often have raised inflammatory markers, e.g. C-reactive protein, which reflect disease activity and help to monitor treatment. Bone erosions can be seen on X-ray. The management of RA requires a multidisciplinary team approach. Treatment aims at relieving joint pain and swelling, preventing structural damage and deformity and minimising disability.

Treatment

Symptom modifying drugs, such as non-steroidal anti-inflammatory drugs (NSAIDs) provide rapid improvement in joint pain and swelling. Disease modifying antirheumatic drugs (DMARDs) delay and may prevent disease progression and joint erosion. They are slow acting (six weeks to six months) and potentially toxic and therefore require close monitoring. They include methotrexate, gold salts, penicillamine, leflunomide, cyclosporin, cyclophosphamide, corticosteroids (oral and intra-articular), infliximab (a monoclonal antibody against TNF) and etanercept (recombinant-soluble TNF receptor).

Some drugs have oral side effects, e.g. mouth ulcers with methotraxate and gold salts. Joint surgery is helpful to alleviate pain and improve function in patients with irreversible joint damage and can be arthroplasty (joint replacement) or arthrodesis (joint fusion).

Other connective tissue diseases

Connective tissue diseases (collagen vascular diseases) are multi-system disorders characterised by pathological changes in blood vessels and connective tissue. The spectrum of disease presentation and severity is wide. Constitutional symptoms such as malaise, tiredness, fever and weight loss are common in all the connective tissue diseases, especially in the acute phase.

Systemic lupus erythematosus

In systemic lupus erythematosus (SLE) any organ may be involved with variable severity. In the acute phase, patients may have a malar butterfly rash on the face (see Colour Plate 11) with arthropathy, serositis, glomerulonephritis or neuropsychiatric manifestations. The oral ulcers occur as painless discrete ulcers often on the hard palate and gingivitis is seen. In discoid LE lesions may appear on the buccal mucosa or as discrete white patches similar to lichen planus. Early and effective immunosuppressive treatment is mandatory.

Dermatomyositis and systemic sclerosis

In dermatomyositis (DM) the main inflammatory impact is against skeletal muscle resulting in muscle weakness of trunk and limbs but respiratory muscle weakness can occur. There is often an erythematous rash on the face and backs of the hands. Pulmonary fibrosis is common.

Systemic sclerosis

In progressive systemic sclerosis (PSS) or scleroderma, diffuse thickening of the skin due to increased collagen deposition and fibrosis occurs and internal organs such as the heart, lungs, kidney and bowel may be involved. Tightening of facial skin may result in difficulty with mouth opening (microstomia) which may cause problems when undertaking dental treatment.

Wegener's granulomatosis

Wegener's granulomatosis is characterised by aggressive tissue necrosis in midline structures such as the nose, sinuses and oral mucosa. Typically ulceration and secondary sepsis with granuloma formation occur. Patients may have an unpleasant nasal discharge but they may present to the dentist with extensive mouth ulceration, gingivitis and foetor.

Rare rheumatological conditions

In **polyarteritis nodosa** small and medium-sized arteries are involved with inflammation of the vessel wall leading to tissue damage and organ infarction, e.g. of the lungs or kidneys. In **giant cell arteritis** localised inflammation of cranial arteries occurs causing unilateral headache, scalp tenderness, facial pain, claudication of the muscles of mastication and blindness due to involvement of the retinal artery.

Behcet's disease is a rare rheumatic condition that may present to the dentist with superficial or deep painful mouth ulcers. Genital ulceration, arthropathy, spondylitis, uveitis, vasculitis and bowel disease are other features. In all these disorders prompt assessment and referral to specialists can result in rapid improvement and may be life-saving.

Sjogren's syndrome and dry mouth

Dry mouth is commonly due to Sjogren's syndrome, a slowly progressive, autoimmune inflammatory disorder of exocrine glands in which the glands are infiltrated by lymphocytes that cause destruction. The salivary glands may initially be enlarged, but later become atrophic. Other organs affected include nasal and bronchial mucosa, vaginal mucosa and lacrimal glands (causing dry, irritable red eyes).

Symptoms

Dry mouth or xerostomia results from a reduction in saliva production from the salivary glands. Patients have difficulty chewing and swallowing their food due to decreased lubrication. They also report problems articulating words, with alteration of taste, discomfort with dentures and difficulty maintaining dental hygiene. Sometimes they report a sore 'burning' mouth. The impaired oral hygiene brings with it a higher risk of dental caries.

Examination of the mouth reveals a dry mouth and tongue with scanty, sticky saliva. There may be erythema of the oral mucosa and reduced numbers of filiform papillae on the tongue, giving a smooth, atrophic appearance (atrophic glossitis). The salivary glands may be palpable in some cases.

Associated conditions

Sjogren's syndrome may be primary occurring on its own or secondary when associated with connective tissue disorder, e.g. RA, SLE, PSS and DM. When assessing a patient with dry mouth one should enquire about symptoms of connective tissue disorders. Patients with Sjogren's syndrome may also have Raynaud's phenomenon, interstitial lung disease, autoimmune liver disease and interstitial nephritis.

Diagnosis

Most patients with secondary Sjogren's syndrome are women (F:M 9:1) with symptoms evolving in the fourth or fifth decade. Apart from dry eyes and dry mouth, examination may reveal rheumatoid arthritis or a connective tissue disorder. Blood tests may reveal anaemia, raised C-reactive protein or a specific autoantibody profile (e.g. a positive DNA antibody test as in SLE).

Tests of salivary gland function include measurement of saliva production, sialography (cannulation of the salivary duct with injection of contrast dye to outline the gland), scintigraphy using radioisotopes to highlight inflammation in salivary glands and salivary gland biopsy. A biopsy of a labial gland, just inside the mouth, may be sufficient to confirm the lymphocytic infiltrate.

Treatment

Treatment is directed at the use of artificial tears or artificial saliva, stimulation of residual salivary function with sugar-free lozenges, attention to mouth, dental and gum hygiene (regular input from dentist and dental hygienist) and the avoidance of smoking. Any associated rheumatic disorder should be appropriately treated. Drugs with an anticholinergic effect, e.g. phenothiazines, antidepressants and antiparkinsonian drugs, tend to make dry mouth worse and their use may need to be modified.

Mouth ulcers, dental care and rheumatic diseases

Mouth ulcers are a common feature of many rheumatic disorders, either due to the inflammatory process affecting the mouth or due to toxicity of medications.

Rheumatic causes of mouth ulceration

Patients with RA frequently complain of superficial aphthous ulceration. It is usually mild but occasionally chronic. In inflammatory bowel disease mouth ulceration (and arthropathy) may occur. Similarly, in Reiter's disease, characterised by arthritis, non-specific urethritis and conjunctivitis, painful and sometimes extensive mouth ulceration is seen. SLE, polyarteritis nodosa, Wegener's granulomatosis, DM and Behcet's disease can all cause mouth ulceration, sometimes with deep scarring ulcers, due to vasculitis with local mucosal necrosis.

Drug-induced oral ulceration

NSAID gold, D-penicillamine, salazopyrin, methotrexate, azathioprine and cyclophosphamide can all cause mouth ulcers which are usually mild and improves on drug withdrawal. Hydrocortisone pellets (Corlan), or stronger steroids such as Adcortyl in Orabase are useful treatments. Tetracycline, hydrocortisone or chlorhexidine mouthwashes may also help.

Parotid gland enlargement

Massive parotid gland enlargement is uncommon in secondary Sjogren's syndrome but may be seen as a slowly evolving enlargement in primary Sjogren's syndrome (when it can be complicated by bacterial infection). Unilateral swelling may be due to neoplasm, e.g. lymphoma or a blocked salivary duct leading to chronic sialadenitis. Bilateral enlargement of parotid glands occurs in acute viral infections, e.g. mumps and Epstein–Barr virus, in sarcoidosis and rarely in diabetes.

Table 15.1 Oral manifestations of rheumatic conditions

Condition	Manifestation
rheumatoid arthritis (RA)	aphthous mouth ulceration occurring spontaneously or secondary to anti-inflammatory or second line suppressive drugs, particularly gold, penicillamine or methotrexate dry mouth due to secondary Sjogren's syndrome temporomandibular joint inflammation or articular damage. Under-development of the jaw in juvenile chronic arthritis causing micrognathia pain originating from the neck due to subluxation at the atlanto-axial joint or subaxial levels causing neck pain, limitation of movement, instability and potentially neurological deficit functional difficulties due to extensive upper limb arthritis causing difficulty brushing and maintaining good dental hygiene
ankylosing spondylitis	progressive spinal inflammation with ankylosis of spinal joints patients may have a very stiff neck with difficulty getting the neck into a suitable examination position
progressive systemic sclerosis (PSS)	difficulty opening the mouth with microstomia and gaining access for dental treatment due to tightening of the mouth xerostomia due to secondary Sjogren's syndrome. May lack dexterity for dental hygiene due to tight contractures of the fingers
systemic lupus erythematosus (SLE)	painless discrete ulcers often on the hard palate. Discoid lupus causes ulcers in buccal mucosa xerostomia due to secondary Sjogren's syndrome
polymyositis (PM)	if severe may cause difficulty maintaining head and neck control due to muscle weakness xerostomia due to secondary Sjogren's syndrome
Behcet's syndrome	deep, painful, scarring mouth ulcers
Wegener's granulomatosis (WG)	deep painful necrotic mouth ulcers with gingivitis secondary bacterial infection $\pm$ candidiasis intense immunosuppression in treated patients may complicate local infection may have nasal and sinus complications from midline granulomatous disease
polyarteritis nodosa (PAN)	may have mouth ulcers due to vasculitis secondary Sjogren's syndrome causing dry mouth

Bacteraemia and joint sepsis

Bacteria from teeth and gums may produce a bacteraemia that can result in infection of joints previously damaged from arthritis or of artificially replaced joints. Patients with joint replacements may require cover with an antibiotic for dental work.

Facial pain and neck instability

Facial pain can result from referred toothache, from TMJ involvement or malocclusion, or may be caused by temporal or giant cell arteritis with pain occurring on mastication due to muscle ischaemia. It is unusual for facial pain to be referred from the neck. Subluxation of the neck in rheumatoid arthritic patients is a risk during intubation for general anaesthesia and it is important not to manipulate the neck into abnormal positions when the neck is unstable. Patients with ankylosing spondylitis may have a very stiff, almost rigid neck.

Disability and mobility

Two of the biggest problems for patients with a severe deforming arthropathy of the upper limbs are maintaining adequate dental hygiene and mobility problems getting to a dentist. Physiotherapists and occupational therapists can help improve function and mobility.

Summary: rheumatological diseases

The oral manifestations of rheumatic conditions are shown in Table 15.1.

References

Moutsopaulos, H.M., Talal, N. (1989) New developments in Sjogren's syndrome. *Curr Opin Rheumatol* 1, 332–8.
Snaith, M.L. (2001) *ABC of Rheumatology*. 2nd edition. London, BMJ Publishing.

Websites

American College of Rheumatology: http://www.rheumatology.org/
Arthritis and Rheumatism Council: http://www.arc.org.uk/

CHAPTER 16
Psychiatric Diseases

This chapter outlines the work of the psychiatrist and describes the presenting features of the major categories of illness met in psychiatry. It includes a table of the main psychopharmacological groups, their indications and side effects.

The role of the psychiatrist

Psychiatrists have trained as medical doctors before choosing to specialise in the diagnosis and treatment of mental health problems. Treatments can be categorised in three ways: biological, psychological and social. Biological treatments include the use of drugs and electro-convulsive therapy (ECT).

Psychological treatments are numerous but examples are behavioural and psychoanalytical therapies. An example of a social treatment is the self-help group. The major categories of illness in psychiatry are dementia and delirium, substance misuse disorders, schizophrenia, depression and mania, and anxiety disorders.

Some other psychiatric conditions can have an impact on the dentist, e.g. in patients with anorexia nervosa and bulimia who induce vomiting, tooth enamel may be damaged by stomach acid.

Dementia and delirium

Dementia is a global impairment of brain function rather than simply a memory problem. Other features that may be present include difficulties with language, poor recognition of faces and places, changes in behaviour, hallucinations, rigidity and incontinence. It is usually a chronic, persistent and progressive condition.

Initially most sufferers have normal concentration and attention. The prevalence in the population aged over 65 is about 5%. The dental practitioner will see more cases in the future as the population proportion over this age increases. Alzheimer's disease is the most common cause.

Delirium can be confused with dementia. There are many causes such as infection, metabolic disturbance, brain insult and anoxia. It has an acute onset and fluctuating symptoms with a typically short course. Compare this with dementia as described above. The cardinal feature is impairment of consciousness. This can range from mild in nature, involving changes in attention and understanding, to extreme such as coma. The patient can be drowsy or hypervigilant, paranoid, and hallucinated. The symptoms may change within hours and are characteristically worse at night.

Substance misuse disorders

Drug abuse is a vague term best avoided. Harmful use of a drug is defined as a pattern of drug use which damages physical, mental or social health. Drug dependence involves both a psychological element, such as a craving, and a physical element such as a withdrawal state.

Other features of dependence include tolerance, neglect of other interests, a stereotyped pattern of drug taking and rapid relapse into dependence following an abstinence period. Substances used in our society are either legal or illegal. Legal substances include alcohol, nicotine and caffeine. Illegal ones include cannabis, LSD, ecstasy, amphetamine and heroin.

Between 5 and 10% of the UK population may have alcohol dependence. An individual who is dependent on alcohol frequently suffers a withdrawal prodrome after approximately 6–12 hours following a significant drop in blood alcohol levels. Features of this prodrome include tremor, sweating, palpitations, nausea and anxiety. These features are usually relieved by resumption of alcohol intake.

In about 20% of individuals with dependence on alcohol, this prodrome can be followed by seizures and a confusional state known as delirium tremens (DTs). The peak period for the onset of DTs is between 48–72 hours. Aside from the typical features of a delirium, DTs classically present with frightening visual hallucinations, usually of small animals, spiders or small people. The mortality rate is around 5%.

Heroin use and dependence is a major medical and social problem in the UK. The drug may be snorted, smoked in a cigarette, inhaled on a heated foil, or injected, usually into a vein. Dependence usually requires daily administration of the drug for at least several weeks.

Features of intoxication include pinpoint pupils, sedation and euphoria. Features of withdrawal may be mild, including yawning, rhinorrhoea and dilated pupils, or more severe where an individual might report muscle cramps, diarrhoea and marked agitation. The withdrawal is very unpleasant but not life-threatening. Amphetamine and cocaine are both stimulants. Ecstasy has some amphetamine-like properties but also induces a sense of well being.

Schizophrenia

This is not a 'split personality'. It has a lifetime prevalence of 1% in the population, usually with its onset in young adults. There is strong evidence for a neurodevelopment aetiology and environmental factors are important. It can be most simply understood as a disorder with two symptom profiles: positive and negative features.

Positive features include delusions, hallucinations, passivity and thought disorder. Negative features most often occur when the schizophrenia is chronic and includes apathy, social withdrawal, and limited ideas in the speech content.

Delusions are fixed, false ideas which are outside the believer's culture and not amenable to reasoning. There are many types: delusions of persecution, wealth, and power are but some. An example of a persecutory delusion is where a man believes that his 90-year-old neighbour is trying to kill him with an X-ray machine.

Hallucinations are perceptions without any external source. They can occur in any of the sensory modalities but are most often auditory. Voices can be derogatory or can command the individual to do something.

Passivity occurs where an individual believes that something outside of himself is affecting his thoughts or actions. Thought disorder is a remarkable sign. It occurs where ideas or even words are not linked together in their usual way resulting in confusion for the listener.

Depression and mania

Mood describes a sustained state of emotions in relation to the surroundings. In depression the mood is usually sad but can be apathetic. Other key features include a decrease in energy levels and a loss of enjoyment in activities that would usually be pleasurable.

We all experience some of these features from time to time but in depression the low mood is sustained and disabling to some degree.

In mania the mood is elevated out of keeping with environmental factors and is sustained.

When an individual is depressed the sleep, appetite, weight and sex drive may be affected. The thoughts become dark and hopeless and suicidal urges may be present. Drug treatments are shown in Table 16.1. In mania the individual has increased energy levels and may behave in ways which involve risk taking and poor judgement such as dangerous driving and inappropriate sexual advances. A medical problem may be the cause of the mood disturbance in both depression and mania. Neurological disorders with endocrine problems are well-known causes. Medication such as steroids can also drastically affect mood.

Anxiety

Anxiety has three components. The first is a sense of apprehension. This can show itself as worrying about the future and difficulties in concentrating. The second consists of motor tension, which is often seen as tremor and fidgeting. The third is autonomic overactivity exemplified by palpitations, butterflies in the stomach and shortness of breath.

If anxiety is only experienced in certain situations then it is a phobia. Common phobias include heights, spiders and going to the dentist. If it occurs out of the blue and leads to a fear of dying or of passing out then the individual suffers from panic disorder. If it present for most of the time and is disabling then it is a generalised anxiety disorder.

Dental phobia is very common. It is best managed by a behavioural treatment called graded exposure. A sufferer starts by building up a hierarchy of stages that would normally produce increasing levels of anxiety. As the individual copes with exposure to a particular stage he or she goes up to the next stage. The last stage might be to sit in a dentist's chair. The lowest might be to look at the chair in a magazine.

Summary: Psychological diseases

- **Dementia** is a chronic and progressive global impairment of brain function that may give problems with memory and behaviour.
- **Delirium** is a condition of impaired consciousness that may be caused by metabolic or infective problems.
- **Substance abuse disorder** represents harmful use of a drug and has a psychological element. Alcohol dependency is found in 5–10% of UK residents.

Table 16.1 The main drugs used for psychiatric treatments and their side effects

Type of drug	Examples	Main indications	Side effects
Antidepressants			
tricyclics	amitriptyline, imipramine	depression	anticholinergic, nausea, sedation, cardiotoxic in overdose
selective serotonin re-uptake inhibitors (SSRIs)	fluoxetine (Prozac) paroxetine	depression, panic disorder	sexual dysfunction, gastrointestinal disturbance
Antipsychotics			
'typical'	chlorpromazine haloperidol thioridazine	schizophrenia, mania	extra pyramidal effects, anti-cholinergic, sedation, weight gain
'atypical'	risperidone, olanzapine	schizophrenia	much lower incidence of the side effects than for 'typicals'
Anxiolytics			
benzodiazepines	diazepam, temazepam	severe anxiety and insomnia, (short term only) alcohol withdrawal	addictive
beta blockers	propranolol	physical manifestations of anxiety	cardiac effects, e.g. bradycardia, bronchospasm
Mood stabiliser			
lithium		treatment of, and prophylaxis in, mania	short term include tremor, metallic taste, weight gain long term include hypothyroidism and renal impairment. toxicity occurs above a set range with marked tremor, vomiting and diarrhoea, thirst, cerebellar signs, rigidity and coma

- **Schizophrenia** is a complex condition with delusions, hallucinations, apathy and social withdrawal.
- **Depression** is a sustained state of sadness in which the patient's sleep, appetite, weight and sex drive may be affected.
- **Mania** is characterised by increased energy levels, risk taking and behaviour showing poor judgement.
- **Anxiety** is a disorder of apprehension, motor tension and autonomic overactivity (e.g. butterflies in the stomach).
- **Dental phobia** is common and best treated by the behaviour treatment of graded exposure.

Further reading

Gelder, M. (ed) (1996) *The Oxford Textbook of Psychiatry*. 3rd edition. Oxford, Oxford University Press.

Website

Royal College of Psychiatrists: http://www.rcpsych.ac.uk

CHAPTER 17
Pregnancy

Pregnancy is the most common reason for absence of menstruation in women of reproductive age (15–44 years). Before embarking on dental treatment, the possibility of pregnancy should be considered. Dental practice should be modified in pregnancy to take account of maternal physiological changes and the susceptibility of the developing fetus to medications administered to its mother.

Physiological changes in the oral cavity with pregnancy

Pregnancy is associated with physiological changes in the oral cavity. Pregnancy gingivitis is seen when the rise in hormone levels in pregnancy appears to influence gingival tissues, resulting in an increased prevalence and severity of gingivitis. The condition increases in severity up to the last 4–6 weeks of pregnancy and then regresses postpartum. Symptoms and complications can be minimised by attention to oral hygiene.

Hormone-induced increased vascularity in an area of plaque stagnation or irritation contributes to a granulomatous/fibrotic response characteristic of a pregnancy epulis. About 1% of pregnant women are affected. Removal is often followed by recurrence and thus treatment should be deferred until after delivery.

Modification of dental treatment

In pregnancy dental treatment requires modification because of the progressive increase in the size of the uterus and physiological changes in maternal respiratory, cardiovascular, gastrointestinal and haematological systems, and because drugs and X-rays used in dental treatment may adversely affect the developing foetus.

Elective dental procedures can be postponed until postpartum. Necessary procedures should be performed during the second trimester (weeks 14–28). By 14 weeks organogenesis is complete and the period of maximum risk of spontaneous miscarriage is over. In the third trimester (weeks 29–40), growth of the foetus makes it difficult for the mother to lie comfortably in one position for any length of time and she may experience supine hypotension syndrome.

Physiological changes in pregnancy

Respiratory and cardiovascular systems

At least 50% of pregnant women experience a sensation of breathlessness. There is no physiological basis for this. Cardiac output rises by 30–50% during pregnancy. Heart rate rises by about 10 beats per minute. Pregnant women may feel lightheaded or faint if they lie on their back. This phenomenon, known as supine hypotensive syndrome, is due to venocaval compression by the pregnant uterus (Figure 17.1). Reduced maternal cardiac output predisposes to a reduction in placental perfusion which can adversely affect foetal well being.

Haematological system

Plasma volume increases in pregnancy by 50% but red blood cell mass increases by only 20–25%. This results in a dilutional anaemia which is maximal around 32 weeks of pregnancy.

Iron deficiency anaemia is the commonest non-physiological cause for anaemia and mainly occurs in the third trimester. Pregnancy

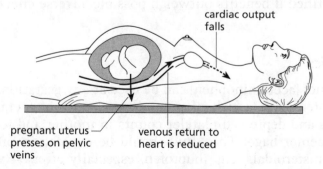

cardiac output
falls

pregnant uterus
presses on pelvic
veins

venous return to
heart is reduced

Figure 17.1 Supine hypotensive syndrome.

is associated with an increase in many of the blood clotting factors. The risk of venous thromboembolism increases especially in the puerperium (6–8 weeks postpartum).

Gastrointestinal system

Compared with non-pregnant women, pregnant women have lower intraoesophageal pressures, higher intragastric pressures and delayed gastric emptying. They are more likely to experience gastro-oesophageal reflux and vomiting – both may adversely affect dental hygiene and contribute to enamel erosion.

Use of drugs for dental treatment in pregnancy

Almost any drug given to the mother will cross the placenta and reach the fetal circulation. Teratogenic risk to the fetus is maximal during organogenesis. This is complete by the end of the first trimester. Drugs given later in pregnancy are not free from foetal effects and the decision to medicate should always be a balance between foetal risk and maternal benefit.

Antimicrobials

Penicillin, cephalosporins and clindamycin can be used throughout pregnancy. Erythromycin is a suitable alternative for penicillin sensitive women, but avoid the estolate form if possible as it is hepatotoxic in some women. Avoid metronidazole in the first trimester. Tetracycline should not be given in pregnancy as it causes staining of teeth and bones. Nystatin may be used at all gestations to treat oral candidiasis. Miconazole and amphotericin should be avoided. Aciclovir has been used in pregnancy to treat genital herpes, HIV infection and other life-threatening viral infections, e.g. chickenpox pneumonia. Its safety is not proven but its use is justified if benefits outweigh possible adverse effects on the fetus.

Analgesics

Paracetamol (acetaminophen) can be used at any gestation. Aspirin is associated with a risk of premature closure of foetal ductus arteriosus and depressed platelet counts in mother and fetus with risk of haemorrhage. This drug should be avoided in pregnancy. Avoid non-steroidals, e.g. ibuprofen, especially after 34 weeks. If given, administer only acutely, i.e. no longer than 24 hours, as there are concerns about premature closure of fetal ductus arteriosus. Avoid sedatives and hypnotics. Entonox (nitrous oxide/oxygen mixture) may be used for 20–30 minutes to provide sedation for anxious women.

Amalgam

Although in theory there is no restriction on use of mercury amalgam, in practice it is not recommended.

Anaesthetics

Local anaesthetics (lignocaine and prilocaine) may be used at all gestations. The combination of local anaesthetic with adrenaline is considered safe, but local anaesthetic combined with vasopressin should be avoided.

General anaesthesia should be avoided. Its use is associated with a risk of preterm delivery and maternal inhalation and aspiration syndrome. If general anaesthesia is unavoidable it should be confined to the second trimester and administered by an obstetric anaesthetist.

X-rays

The dose of radiation from dental X-rays is very small – chest X-ray results in 800 times estimated fetal exposure to radiation compared with full mouth dental series (18 intraoral radiographs, D film, lead apron). However, avoid X-rays in the first trimester unless absolutely essential and obtain only essential views using a high-speed film, filtration and collimation. The patient should be provided with a protective lead apron to minimise gonadal and fetal exposure.

Dental treatment postpartum

Most physiological changes do not return to the pre-pregnancy state until 4–6 weeks postdelivery. During this period dental treatment should be as for the pregnant woman.

Breastfeeding needs to be considered. The transfer of most drugs in breast milk is minimal and for many medications breastfeeding can be continued. Advise taking any medication just after breastfeeding if possible, to minimise neonatal exposure. Indomethacin, penicillin and metronidazole may be administered to breastfeeding women. Aspirin and tetracycline should be avoided.

Summary: Pregnancy

- **Avoid stress** and provide reassurance – women are often worried about any therapy in pregnancy. Treat infection and/or pain.
- **Encourage good dental hygiene** and use dental sessions as an opportunity to educate about infant dental care and diet.
- **First and third trimesters** – limit treatment to necessary minimum. Avoid procedures longer than 20 minutes until at least three months postpartum.
- **Second trimester** – give routine care.
- **Avoid X-rays** unless essential and restrict prescription drugs to those known to be safe in pregnancy.
- **Carefully document** all investigations performed and treatment plan – with explanations.

Further reading

Tilakaratne, A., Soory, M., Ranasinghe, A.W., Corea, S.M.X., Ekanayake, S.L., De Silva, M. (2000) Periodontal disease status during pregnancy and three months postpartum in a rural population of Sri Lankan women. *J Clin Periodontol* 2000, 27, 722–32.

Soory, M. (2000) Hormonal factors in periodontal disease. *Dental Update* 27, 380–83.

Lee, A., McWilliams, M., Janchar, T. (1999) Care of the pregnant dental patient in the dental office. *Dent Clin North Am* 43, 485–94.

Department of Health (1998) *Statement on the toxicity of dental amalgam*. London, Department of Health.

Websites

Pregnancy gingivitis: http://www.dentistry.com/pbrightersmile_03.asp
Dental amalgam: http://www.doh.gov.uk/hef/amalgam.htm

CHAPTER 18

Accident and Emergency Medicine

The dentist will have to deal with medical emergencies from time to time. These may take the form of a sudden collapse, e.g. from an acute myocardial infarction, or from a head injury. This chapter outlines the clinical management of these important medical emergencies.

Cardiopulmonary resuscitation

The purpose of cardiopulmonary resuscitation is to maintain adequate ventilation and circulation until means can be obtained to reverse the underlying cause of the arrest. It is therefore a 'holding operation', although on occasions, particularly when the primary disease is respiratory failure, it may itself reverse the cause and allow full recovery.

Consequences of circulatory failure

Failure of the circulation for 3–4 minutes (less if the patient is initially hypoxaemic) will lead to irreversible cerebral damage. Delay, even within that time, will lessen the eventual chances of a successful outcome. Emphasis must therefore be placed on rapid institution of basic life support by a rescuer, who should follow the recommended sequence of action.

Basic life support

Basic life support (BLS) comprises:
- initial assessment
- airway maintenance

- expired air ventilation ('rescue breathing')
- chest compression.

When all are combined the term 'cardiopulmonary resuscitation' (CPR) is used. Basic life support implies that no equipment is employed; where a simple airway or facemask for mouth-to-mouth ventilation is used, this is defined as 'basic life support with airway adjunct'. The three elements of basic life support after initial assessment are commonly remembered as 'A–B–C': Airway–Breathing–Circulation.

Sequence of actions

1. **Ensure safety** of rescuer and victim.
2. **Check the victim** and see if he responds: Gently shake his shoulders and ask loudly: 'Are you all right?'
3a. **If he responds** by answering or moving:
    - Leave him in the position in which you find him (provided he is not in further danger), check his condition and get help if needed.
    - Reassess him regularly.
3b. **If he does not respond:**
    - Shout for help.
    - Unless you can assess him fully in the position you find him, turn the victim on to his back and then open the airway. (Figure 18.1).
        - Place your hand on his forehead and gently tilt his head back keeping your thumb and index finger free to close his nose if rescue breathing is required.
        - Remove any visible obstruction from the victim's mouth, including dislodged dentures, but leave well-fitting dentures in place.
        - With your fingertip(s) under the point of the victim's chin, lift the chin to open the airway.
Try to avoid head tilt if trauma (injury) to the neck is suspected
4. Keeping the airway open, **look, listen and feel** for breathing (more than an occasional gasp or weak attempts at breathing):

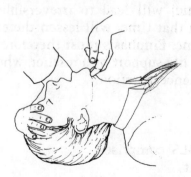

Figure 18.1 Open the airway by head tilt/chin lift.

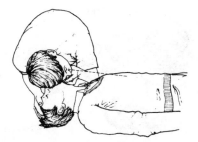

Figure 18.2 Look, listen and feel for breathing.

    – Look for chest movement.
    – Listen at the victim's mouth for breath sounds.
    – Feel for air on your cheek.
   • Look, listen and feel for no more than 10 seconds to determine if the victim is breathing normally (Figure 18.2).

5a. If he is breathing normally:
   • Turn him into the recovery position.
   • Send or go for help.
   • Check for continued breathing.

5b. If he is not breathing, or is only making occasional gasps or weak attempts at breathing:
   • Send someone for help or, if you are on your own, leave the victim and go for help: return and start rescue breathing as below
   • Turn the victim onto his back if he is not already in this position
   • Give two slow, effective rescue breaths, each of which makes the chest rise and fall
    – Ensure head tilt and chin lift.
    – Pinch the soft part of his nose closed with the index finger and thumb of your hand on his forehead (Figure 18.3a).
    – Open his mouth a little, but maintain chin lift.
    – Take a deep breath and place your lips around his mouth, making sure that you have a good seal.

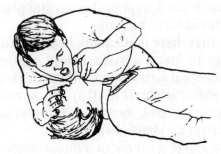

Figure 18.3a Ensure head tilt/chin lift, pinch the nose.

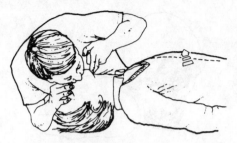

Figure 18.3b Blow steadily into the mouth, watching for the chest to rise.

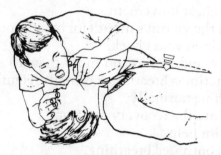

Figure 18.3c Watch for the chest to fall as air comes out.

    – Blow steadily into his mouth whilst watching his chest; take about 2 seconds to make his chest rise as in normal breathing (Figure 18.3b).

    – Maintain head tilt and chin lift, take your mouth away from the victim and watch for his chest to fall as air comes out (Figure 18.3c).

- Take another breath and repeat the sequence as above to give two effective rescue breaths in all

- If you have difficulty achieving an effective breath:

    – **Recheck the victim's mouth** for any evidence of secretions, blood, vomitus or other potential materials that might be causing acute airways obstruction. You may need to immediately apply suction or finger sweeps to remove the material to clear a potential or actual occlusion and prevent aspiration of foreign material into the lungs.

    – **Recheck that there is adequate head tilt and chin lift**. It may be necessary to insert a basic airway adjunct (oropharyngeal or nasopharyngeal airway) to maintain airway control.

    – Make up to five attempts in all to achieve two effective breaths.

    – Even if unsuccessful, move on to assessment of circulation.

6.   Assess the person for **signs of circulation**:

- Look, listen and feel for normal breathing, coughing or movement by the victim.

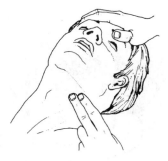

Figure 18.4 Feel the carotid pulse.

- **Only if you have been trained to do so**, check the carotid pulse (Figure 18.4).
- Take no more than 10 seconds to do this.

7a. If you are confident that you can detect signs of a circulation:
- Continue rescue breathing until the victim starts breathing on his own.
- About every 10 breaths (or about every minute) recheck for signs of a circulation; take no more than 10 seconds each time.
- If the victim starts to breathe on his own but remains unconscious, turn him into the recovery position. Be ready to turn him onto his back and re-start rescue breathing if he stops breathing.

7b. If there are no signs of a circulation, or you are at all unsure:
- Start chest compression:
  - With your hand that is nearer the victim's feet, locate the lower half of the sternum.
  - Using your index and middle fingers, identify the lower rib margins. Keeping your finders together, slide them upwards to the point where the ribs join the sternum. With your middle finger on this point, place your index finger on the sternum.
  - Slide the heel of your other hand down the sternum until it reaches your index finger; this should be the middle of the lower half of the sternum (Figure 18.5).

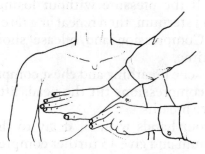

Figure 18.5 Locate the middle of the lower half of the sternum.

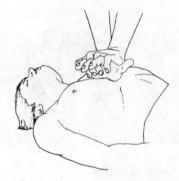

Figure 18.6 Interlock the fingers of both hands and lift them to ensure pressure is not applied over the victim's ribs.

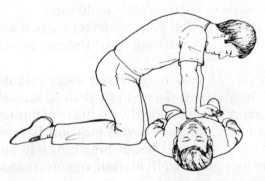

Figure 18.7 Position yourself vertically above the victim.

– Place the heel of the other hand on top of the first.
– Extend or interlock the fingers of both hands and lift them to ensure that pressure is not applied over the victim's ribs. Do not apply any pressure over the upper abdomen or bottom tip of the sternum (Figure 18.6).
– Position yourself vertically above the victim's chest and, with your arms straight, press down on the sternum to depress it between 4–5 cm (Figure 18.7).
– Release all the pressure without losing contact between the hand and sternum, then repeat at a rate of about 100 times a minute. Compression and release should take an equal amount of time.
• Combine rescue breathing and chest compression:
– After 15 compressions tilt the head, lift the chin and give two effective breaths
– Return your hands without delay to the correct position on the sternum and give 15 further compressions, continuing compressions and breaths in a ratio of 15:2.

8.   **Continue resuscitation until**:
     – qualified help arrives and takes over
     – the victim shows signs of life
     – you become exhausted.

When to go for assistance

It is vital for rescuers to get help as quickly as possible. When more than one rescuer is available, one should start resuscitation while another rescuer goes for help.

A single rescuer will have to decide whether to start resuscitation or to go for help first. If the victim is an adult, the single rescuer should normally assume that he has a heart problem and go for help immediately it has been established he is not breathing. This decision may be influenced by the availability of emergency medical services.

However, if the likely cause of unconsciousness is a breathing problem, as in:

• trauma
• drowning
• choking
• drug or alcohol intoxication
• or if the victim is an infant or child

The rescuer should perform resuscitation for about one minute before going for help.

Resuscitation with two persons

It is recommended that only trained healthcare providers use this technique. A ratio of 15 chest compressions to two inflations should be used (Figure 18.8).

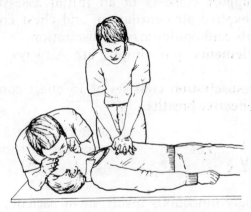

Figure 18.8 Resuscitation with two persons.

Precautions

Cross-infection between victim and rescuer potentially may occur during mouth-to-mouth ventilation. The incidence is remarkably rare but isolated cases of cutaneous tuberculosis, herpes labialis, staphylococcal and streptococcal infections and meningococcal meningitis have been reported. Of great concern to would-be rescuers is the possibility of acquiring human immunodeficiency virus (HIV) during mouth-to-mouth contact. Fortunately it appears that HIV is not contained in saliva in amounts sufficient to cause infection (Centers for Disease Control, 1988) but there always remains the possibility of transmission from open wounds in both parties. There is, however, no record of this occurring at the time of writing and so the possibility must be considered almost negligible. The chance of infection with the hepatitis B virus (HBV) is greater.

Health professionals have a much higher chance of being called upon to perform resuscitation than lay individuals and it is therefore reasonable that protective airway adjuncts should be readily available in each patient area to offer protection against infection and to reduce aesthetic antagonism. The pocket mouth-to-mask device is one of the most satisfactory adjuncts for this purpose.

Summary: Cardiopulmonary resuscitation

• **The purpose of resuscitation** is to maintain ventilation and circulation until means are obtained to reverse the underlying cause of the arrest.
• **Failure of the circulation** for three to four minutes will result in brain damage.
• **Basic life support** consists of an initial assessment, airways maintenance, expired air ventilation, and chest compression: all combined equals cardiopulmonary resuscitation.
• **The three elements**, put simply, are Airways, Breathing and Circulation.
• **Combined resuscitation** consists of 15 chest compressions followed by two effective breaths.

Head injury

After a seemingly innocuous insult, most patients who sustain a head injury recover rapidly and completely, but a significant minority will deteriorate quickly into critical illness demanding immediate intensive care and neurosurgical management.

The spectrum of severity between these extremes underlines the principle that basic, early assessment and simple emergency management of a head injury will optimise the chances of recovery from any brain damage already sustained at the time of injury. Dentists should know the basics of immediate care.

Mechanisms of head injury

Injuries to the facial skeleton and skull vault are significant only in relation to the likelihood of brain damage that they suggest. Head injury severity can be more meaningfully thought of as brain injury severity.

Diffuse brain damage

The spongiform brain is loosely anchored within the rigid skull vault, bathed in a small amount of cerebrospinal fluid (CSF). Strong acceleration or deceleration forces applied to the head, such as occur when the head hits the floor after falling, cause the brain to bang against the bony walls. The brain surface then becomes contused, especially over the frontal and temporal areas where ridges within the cranial cavity tend to catch. Internal shearing forces cause brain tissue to become distorted leading to diffuse axonal injury. Patients with significant diffuse axonal injury may never regain consciousness. In its mildest form, diffuse axonal injury gives rise to concussion where memory lapses, irritability and confusion are self-limiting reflections of mild, recoverable axonal damage.

Focal brain damage

Skull vault fractures: These arise from high-impact blunt forces, e.g. a fall to the floor, or after a blow to the head from a heavy implement. On fracturing, a piece of the skull may be forced inwards, tearing the dura mater. This causes brain distortion and bleeding from superficial vessels. If such a fracture connects to an external wound, then an open depressed skull fracture exists, which is at high risk from infection and urgent neurosurgical debridement is needed.

Extradural haematoma: Following a blunt head injury, transient deformation of the skull may strip off the dura mater creating a

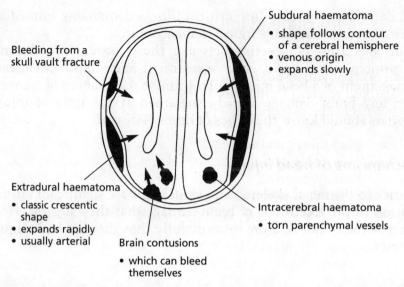

Bleeding from a
skull vault fracture

Subdural haematoma
- shape follows contour
  of a cerebral hemisphere
- venous origin
- expands slowly

Extradural haematoma
- classic crescentic
  shape
- expands rapidly
- usually arterial

Brain contusions
- which can bleed
  themselves

Intracerebral haematoma
- torn parenchymal vessels

Figure 18.9 Brain damage following head injury.

potential space which quickly fills with blood, e.g. from the middle meningeal artery (Figure 18.9). Problems arise when the expanding haematoma compresses the healthy brain tissue. Management aims to minimise the effects of this expansion by relieving pressure, e.g. with craniotomy and clot evacuation.

Intradural haematoma: Bleeding from within the dural layer is more common than extradural bleeding. It arises from torn cerebral veins. Haematoma expansion occurs more slowly than in extradural haematoma and clinical deterioration is more subtle.

There may be no immediate indication that a patient who has fallen and sustained an intradural or subdural haematoma has brain damage at all. They may present days later with progressive drowsiness, nausea, irritability or confusion.

Hypoxic brain damage

An injured brain loses the autoregulatory mechanisms that normally maintain constant brain tissue perfusion, making it susceptible to ischaemic axonal injury, especially if there is other trauma and blood loss. This kind of brain damage is impossible to prevent. Treatment aims to maximise the chances for autoregulation to return, by supplying oxygen and intravenous fluids to the patient and treating other injuries.

Assessment of head injury

Assessment in head-injured patients should identify clinical features which are known to predict an increased risk of significant brain damage, and warrant immediate investigation. In a conversant, conscious patient the essentials are:

Mechanism of injury and acute history: how it happened, the forces involved, was there recollection of events, any witnessed loss of consciousness, vomiting or nausea, ataxia, visual disturbance, drowsiness, slurred speech since the event, or loss of limb function or sensation.

Other relevant factors in individual cases: was any medication normally taken (especially anticoagulants), is the patient diabetic and at risk of hypoglycaemia, is the injury is due to assault which may need to be reported to the police?

Basic management

In a drowsy, unwell patient who has sustained a head injury, the management priorities are to provide a patent, stable airway, to check there is sufficient breathing function and to ensure an adequate circulation. It is usual to prioritise the A–B–C of resuscitation, which applies to all seriously injured patients. Expert help is required immediately in a patient with a head injury who is drowsy or unwell. In a dental practice, this means calling an ambulance at once if serious head injury occurs.

Summary: Head injuries

- Most head injuries are minor and cause minimal physical and emotional sequelae.
- It is important to be able to identify those patients who may have significant brain damage.
- Certain features of the history and examination of the patient help predict these patients.
- Intracranial bleeding is the main cause of the deterioration seen after head injury.
- Patients who take anticoagulants are at greater risk of bleeding after an otherwise minor head injury and must be observed closely.
- Bleeding can occur in various sites within the cranial vault.
- If faced with a drowsy or unwell patient who has sustained a head injury get expert help immediately.

Reference

Centers for Disease Control Update (1988) Universal precautions for prevention of transmission of human immunodeficiency virus, hepatitis B virus and other blood borne pathogens in health care settings. *Morbid Mortal Weekly Rep* 1988, 37, 377–88.

Further reading

Bullock, R., Teasdale, G. (1996) Head Injuries. In Skinner, D., Driscoll, P., Earlam, R. (eds) *ABC of Major Trauma*. 2nd edition, London, BMJ Publishing.
Colquhoun, M.C. (ed) (1999) *ABC of Resuscitation*, 4th edition. London, BMJ Publishing.
Resuscitation Council (UK). Resuscitation Guidelines 2000. London, 2000.

Websites

UK Resuscitation Council: http://www.resus.org.uk
European Resuscitation Council: http://www.erc.edu
British Heart Foundation: http://www.bhf.org.uk
American College of Emergency Physicians: http://www.acep.org

Acknowledgement

Resuscitation guidelines taken, with kind permission, from The Resuscitation Guidelines 2000.

CHAPTER 19

Disability and the Dental Patient

To understand the impact of having a disability, it is important to understand the basic concepts and how to apply these to the real world. The World Health Organization has developed a model of classifying human functioning and disablement called the ICIDH-2 (International Classification of Impairment, Disability and Handicap, 2nd revision).

ICIDH-2 aims to provide a unified language and a framework within which health workers, people with disabilities and others can describe human functioning and disability. Although ICIDH-2 can be useful for scientific purposes, data comparison and audit, in this context it aids communication between our different disciplines (i.e. occupational therapy and dentistry) and provides a framework which will help the dentist to provide non-discriminatory services in the future.

Constraining factors

Impairment represents a problem in body function (physiological or psychological) or in structure such as a significant deviation or loss. This not pathology but how pathology is manifested.

Activities defines the performance of a task or action by an individual. **Limitations** (formerly known as disabilities) are difficulties in the performance of tasks.

Participation includes an individual's involvement in life situations in relation to their health conditions, impairments, activity, environmental and personal factors. It may mean being included in an area of life, being accepted or having access to resources. Environmental factors are the barriers in the environment that restrict participation. Society may hinder participation because it creates barriers, e.g. inaccessible buildings, or because it does not provide facilitators.

Potential problem areas

In a dental practice potential problem areas are:
- **access** to the premises
- **communication** with the staff
- **time** needed for access or treatment (it may be longer)
- **legal responsibilities** for the facilities provided.

Summary: Disability

- **The needs of disabled people** need to be better understood in clinical areas
- **Impaired body functions** may limit the patient's activities
- **Environmental changes** may be needed to reduce barriers, e.g. to improve access to a building
- **Time and communication** are other factors that need to be considered for patients with disability.

Further reading

Demeter, S.L. (1996) *Disability Evaluation*. London, Mosby.

Website

World Health Organization: http://www.who.int

SECTION 3
Pharmacology and Anaesthetics

In most countries dentists prescribe a variety of medications that will include topical agents, e.g. artificial saliva, mouthwashes, oral antifungal and steroid preparations, and topical lidocaine, as well as oral drugs, particularly analgesics, antibiotics, antiherpetic agents, and certain sedatives (e.g. temazepam). Details of these drugs can be found in the readily available general pharmacopoeias, e.g. the *British National Formulary* (which has a *Dental Practitioners' Formulary*).

The purpose of this section to give dentists details of those drugs that they prescribe, and discuss the common types of drugs that their patients' medical practitioners may prescribe. Drug interactions are important and, in order to understand these, some knowledge of the kinetics of drugs is helpful.

CHAPTER 20
Pharmacokinetics and Altered Drug Effects

Pharmacokinetics describes how drugs are processed once they have been delivered to the body and is basic to an understanding of drug prescribing. It can be summarised under the four headings of absorption, distribution, metabolism and elimination. Problems with pharmacokinetics are the commonest reason for withdrawal of a potential new drug during development (followed by lack of efficacy, animal or human toxicity, and other factors).

Routes of drug administration

Drugs may be delivered (Figure 20.1):
- orally – tablet or capsule
- rectally – suppository, enema
- by inhalation to the lungs – inhaler

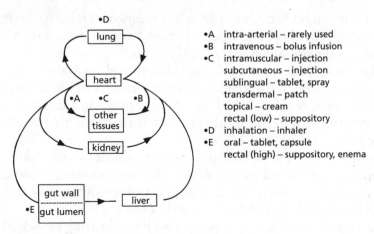

Figure 20.1 Routes of drug administration.

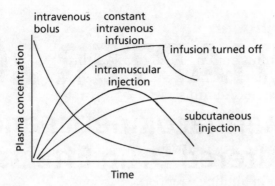

Figure 20.2 Plasma concentrations according to route of drug administration.

- or nose – spray
- sublingually – tablet, spray
- transdermally – patch
- topically – cream, ointment
- subcutaneously – injection
- intralesionally – injection
- intramuscularly – injection
- intravenously – bolus or infusion
- or, rarely, intra-arterially

Whatever the route of administration, drugs may have both local and systemic effects. The concentration of a drug in the plasma rises most rapidly following an intravenous injection. Other routes give a much slower rise and a lower peak level (Figure 20.2). For oral administration, 'sustained-release' preparations give a slower rise but a more sustained level in plasma concentration.

Diffusion and solubility of a drug

To reach its target receptor, a drug has many obstacles to overcome. If delivered via the oral route, it may have to penetrate the gut mucosa, enter the blood via a capillary wall, diffuse into the extra-cellular fluid, penetrate a cell membrane and only then reach the intracellular fluid of its target cell. Drugs usually move across membranes by passive diffusion. The rate of transfer is a function of the concentration difference, multiplied by the surface area, multiplied by the permeability (Fick's law).

Whether or not a drug is lipid or water-soluble is important. Lipid solubility is increased by the drug's chemical structure containing alkyl groups or aromatic rings, whereas water solubility is increased by $-OH$, $-COOH$, and $-NH_2$ groups that show a hydrogen bond. The degree of ionisation of a molecule also has a bearing on whether or not it will penetrate a membrane.

Drug distribution

After oral administration, a drug passes through the gut wall, the hepatic portal vein, the liver, the heart and lungs, only then to enter the arterial system. Administration by any route other than oral will bypass the gut and hence avoid the phenomenon of the 'first-pass' effect of the liver. The distribution of a drug is influenced by:

- **cardiac output** – determines the rate at which a drug is delivered to an organ
- **plasma protein binding** – represents a transport system for drugs
- **lipid solubility** – controls the progress of a drug across a lipid membrane (only non-ionised drugs pass).

The perfusion rate varies widely for different organs, e.g. it is high for the lungs and kidneys, quite high for the liver, heart and brain, and low for other tissues such as fat or muscle. This means that drugs reach a plateau level rapidly in well-perfused organs.

Renal and biliary excretion

The kidneys clear drugs that are water-soluble and ionised, whereas the hepatic route (via the biliary tract) clears drugs that are lipid soluble and non-ionised. The renal clearance is influenced by the rates of filtration and secretion by the kidney minus any reabsorption. The creatinine clearance of the kidneys, a measure of their excretion ability, has a linear effect on the renal excretion of a water-soluble drug eliminated by the renal route.

The pH of the urine also can have an influence. In biliary excretion, seen for polar (ionised) drugs and those with a molecular weight greater then 300 daltons, enterohepatic recycling may prolong the drug effect. In enterohepatic recycling the drug is excreted through the biliary tract only to be reabsorbed from the small bowel (Figure 20.3).

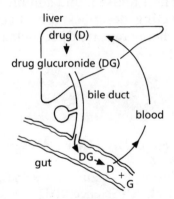

Figure 20.3 Enterohepatic recycling.

Drug metabolism

Several organs can metabolise drugs but the liver is the most important as it is best endowed with microsomal enzymes highly suited to this purpose. Drug metabolism is mainly thought of as a process whereby the drug is deactivated to inactive metabolites without pharmacological effect – but sometimes the process of metabolism actually produces the active substance (as in 'prodrugs').

The biochemical processes of drug metabolism include oxidation, reduction, hydrolysis, glucuronidation, sulphonation, acetylation, methylation and glutathione conjugation. An enzyme system called cytochrome P450 is responsible for some type of drug metabolism. This enzyme system exists in a number of genetic forms or polymorphisms. These are responsible for the variation between individuals in the ability to metabolise drugs. One Caucasian in 12 is a so-called 'poor metaboliser', and these individuals are at higher risk of suffering from drug toxicity.

Summary: Pharmacokinetics

• **Route of administration** of a drug may be oral, rectal, topical, subcutaneous, intravenous, intramuscular or intralesional. The intravenous route results in the most rapid rise in plasma level.
• **Passive diffusion** is the method by which most drugs move across a membrane.
• **Lipid or water solubility** is important: a non-ionised lipid-soluble drug will pass a lipid membrane whereas a water-soluble one will not.
• **The first pass effect** describes when a drug absorbed from the gut is metabolised on the first occasion it moves through the liver before the remainder of it is delivered to the rest of the body.
• **Kidneys** mainly excrete water-soluble ionised drugs, the biliary tract mainly excretes non-ionised lipid-soluble drugs.
• **Enterohepatic recycling** describes the effect whereby a drug's effect is prolonged by being repeatedly recycled through the gut and the hepatobiliary system.

References

Dental Practitioners' Formulary. Updated every two years. London, Pharmaceutical Press.

Reid, J.L., Rubin, P., Whiting, B. *Lecture Notes on Clinical Pharmacology.* 6th edition. Oxford, Blackwell Science, 2001.

Websites

Basic pharmacokinetics:
  http://pharmacy.creighton.edu/pha443/pdf/Default.asp
British National Formulary online: http://www.bnf.org/
Dental Practitioners' Formulary:
  http://www.bnf.org/BNFProductsFrameDPF.htm

CHAPTER 21
Cardiovascular Drugs

The drugs used to treat cardiovascular disease can be divided into those for hypertension, angina, heart failure, acute myocardial infarction and drugs to prevent coronary artery disease (statins and aspirin). In addition, warfarin is given to many cardiac patients, especially those with atrial fibrillation.

Hypertension

Hypertension is very common, affecting 15–20% of adults. The causes and risk factors for high blood pressure are described in Chapter 3, Cardiovascular Diseases. Hypertension is mostly asymptomatic and usually 'idiopathic' (i.e. there is no obvious cause). The rationale for the treatment of hypertension is to prevent the complications that include cerebrovascular disease (stroke), coronary heart disease, left ventricular failure, renal failure and retinopathy.

The successful control of high blood pressure can reduce mortality and morbidity from these complications. The early detection and treatment of hypertension is crucial to reducing complications – safe and long-term therapy is the aim.

Non-pharmacological measures

Some basic lifestyle suggestions may help the hypertensive patient. These include advice to lose weight, take less salt in the diet, reduce alcohol consumption, take more exercise and stop smoking.

Thiazide diuretics

It is usual to initiate treatment of hypertension with a thiazide diuretic such as bendrofluazide. They are inexpensive and have few side effects although they can cause hypokalaemia, gout or hyper-glycaemia. Thiazide diuretics work by increasing salt and water excretion from the kidneys.

Angiotensin converting enzyme (ACE) inhibitors

The ACE inhibitors are effective in hypertension but may initially cause a precipitous fall in the blood pressure. They work by inhibiting the conversion of angiotensin I to angiotensin II.

They are contraindicated in angioedema and hypersensitivity to ACE inhibitors, and when there is suspected renovascular disease or aortic stenosis. Their side effects include renal impairment, a dry cough and altered liver function tests.

Beta blockers

Beta adrenergic blocking agents such as atenolol are commonly used to treat hypertension. They work by reducing cardiac output and by blocking peripheral adrenoreceptors. Beta blockers are contra-indicated in asthma, uncontrolled heart failure and bradycardia. Their side effects include fatigue, hypotension, cold peripheries and bronchospasm.

Calcium channel blockers

Calcium channel blocking agents such as verapamil, amlodipine and nifedipine work as antihypertensive agents by reducing myocardial contractility and systemic vascular tone. Verapamil is contraindicated in heart failure, conduction blocks and with the concomitant use of beta blockers. Amlodipine and nifedipine are contraindicated in aortic stenosis. The side effects include constipation, flushing and headache.

Other drugs

Postsynaptic alpha receptor blocking agents such as prazosin and doxazosin must be used cautiously at first as there can be a large drop in blood pressure after the first dose. The side effects are dizziness, vertigo and fatigue, and a postural drop in blood pressure. Central acting hypotensive agents include methyldopa and clonidine.

Methyldopa has been used to treat hypertension for many years. It is contraindicated in active liver disease and depression. Its side effects include dry mouth, sedation and haemolysis of the red blood cells. Clonidine and moxonidine are occasionally prescribed but care is needed as abrupt withdrawal may lead to rebound hypertension.

Preventive measures in coronary artery disease

Patients with coronary heart disease should be advised to lose weight if obese, to stop smoking, to consume alcohol in moderation (males 21 and females 14 units/week) and to take exercise. If they have diabetes, good control of the blood pressure and sugar is helpful.

If they have elevated serum lipids then control of this hyperlipidaemia with diet and a statin should be considered. Non-steroidal drugs should be avoided as they promote fluid retention that can lead to fluid overload and cardiac failure.

Aspirin

Many patients with coronary artery disease are prescribed aspirin 75 mg once daily. Aspirin works through the thromboxane pathway to prevent platelet aggregation and inhibit thrombus formation. When used for secondary prevention, i.e. after a cardiovascular event has already occurred, aspirin is of proven benefit in the prevention of further vascular disease and in reducing cardiac mortality. Side effects include gastric bleeding.

It is important to stop aspirin a week prior to major dental procedures as the risk of bleeding complications following surgery outweighs benefits. Aspirin can be recommenced postoperatively when it is safe to do so.

Statins

Statins such as simvastatin are a group of drugs used to treat elevated serum levels of cholesterol. They are effective for both the primary and secondary prevention of vascular disease. Hyperlipidaemia is a recognised risk factor for coronary artery disease and its effective treatment is known to reduce cardiac mortality, repeat myocardial infarction (in those who have had a myocardial infarct already), and stroke. The statins work by their effect on a liver enzyme involved in cholesterol synthesis. Side effects include abnormal liver function tests and muscle damage. They are used with caution in patients with liver disease and in those with excessive alcohol intake.

Angina

Myocardial ischaemia due to coronary artery disease is manifest as the chest pain of angina (see Chapter 3, Cardiovascular Diseases).

Patients with angina are assessed for cardiovascular risk factors and given general advice. Several drugs are useful in the management of angina.

Nitrates

Nitrates such as isosorbide mononitrate or glyceryl trinitrate, which may be given in a long-acting form, are useful for the symptomatic relief of angina. They may also be used in heart failure. Nitrates work by producing vasodilation of the coronary arteries but have side effects of headache, flushing and postural hypotension. Nitrates are given by the sublingual or transdermal route for rapid action in acute attacks as they are rapidly metabolised on first pass through the liver. Modified release tablets can be given twice daily. Long-term use leads to tolerance.

Beta blockers

Beta blockers such as atenolol help in angina by reducing the cardiac workload and the risk of cardiac arrhythmias. They improve exercise tolerance and reduce the risk of myocardial infarction. Carvedilol, metoprolol and bisoprolol have been shown to be beneficial in mild to moderate heart failure and can reduce mortality. Side effects include fatigue, hypotension, cold peripheries and bronchospasm. Beta blockers are contraindicated in asthma, uncontrolled heart failure and bradycardia.

Other drugs

Vasodilators such as hydralazine and minoxidil have a direct action as smooth muscle relaxants. Hydralazine is contraindicated in lupus erythematosus, aortic dissection and myocardial insufficiency. Angiotensin II receptor antagonists are a group of drugs similar to the angiotensin converting enzyme inhibitors but they do not give rise to a dry cough as the bradykinin pathway is not affected. Examples include losartan and valsartan. They are contraindicated in renal artery stenosis or renal impairment and in pregnancy.

Calcium channel blockers such as verapamil help by reducing cardiac output and lowering heart rate. Diltiazem, amlodipine and nifedipine work by relaxing vascular smooth muscle tone and dilating the coronary and peripheral arteries. Verapamil, which is contraindicated in heart failure, should not be used with beta blockers.

Heart failure

In heart failure, there is dysfunction of systole and diastole that leads to poor tissue perfusion and elevated filling pressures. This leads to pump failure, with congestion of the lungs, liver and peripheral tissues. Mortality is high. Effective treatment improves symptoms and reduces mortality.

Digoxin

Digoxin is a time-honoured treatment for heart failure and atrial fibrillation. It works by increasing the force of myocardial contraction and by reducing atrioventricular conduction. It is not clear if it has an effect on cardiac mortality. Its therapeutic window is small, i.e. doses that have a therapeutic effect are close to those that cause side effects (which include ventricular arrhythmias, heart block, nausea, fatigue, confusion and altered vision).

Diuretics

Furosemide is a diuretic that works by inhibiting reabsorbtion of sodium in the loop of Henle. Its side effects include low serum potassium and sodium, tinnitus and pancreatitis. Spironolactone is a potassium-sparing diuretic that antagonises aldosterone. It has been shown to have a beneficial effect on cardiac mortality. Its side effects include nausea, gynaecomastia, hyperkaleamia and hyponatraemia. It is contraindicated when there is an elevated serum potassium and in severe renal failure.

Other drugs

Angiotensin converting enzyme (ACE) inhibitors such as captopril, enalapril, lisinopril and ramipril are beneficial in heart failure and have been shown to reduce mortality by 40% over a six-month period. They improve symptoms over the long term.

Potassium channel activating drugs such as nicorandil are used in angina and work by opening the adenosine triphosphate (ATP) sensitive potassium channel in vascular smooth muscle. They are not used in patients who are hypertensive and may have side effects of dizziness and cutaneous vasodilation.

Emergency treatment of acute left ventricular failure

If a patient develops acute left ventricular failure in the ·dentist's surgery, they should be given oxygen by mask, and then transferred by ambulance to an accident and emergency department where, after assessment, they are likely to receive intravenous diamorphine and furosemide. They will then be monitored closely in an intensive care setting and may receive intravenous inotropic agents such as dobutamine.

Acute myocardial infarction

When a patient presents with an acute myocardial infarction, they are given intravenous morphine for pain relief, streptokinase or tissue plasminogen activator for thrombolysis, oxygen, and aspirin for its antithrombotic effect. From the second day onwards, it is common to precribe a beta blocker and ACE inhibitor.

Streptokinase works by inducing the formation of plasmin, a natural thrombolytic agent which dissolves coagulation factors and fibrin clot. Several different type of drug may be used to control arrhythmias, e.g. adenosine, verapamil, beta blockers, disopyramide, flecainide, amiodarone, and mexiletine.

Summary: Cardiovascular drugs

• Table 21.1 summarises the main cardiovascular drugs, their indications and side effects.

Table 21.1 The main drugs used for the treatment of cardiovascular diseases

Drug	Indication	Side effects
thiazide diuretic	first choice for hypertension	hypokalaemia, gout
ACE inhibitor	hypertension, heart failure	cough, renal impairment
beta blocker	hypertension, angina	bronchospasm, fatigue
calcium channel blocker	hypertension, angina	flushing, fluid retention
nitrate	angina, heart failure	headache, flushing
digoxin	heart failure, atrial fibrillation	heart block, nausea
loop diuretic	heart failure	electrolyte imbalance
statin	hypercholesterolaemia	abnormal liver function tests, rhabdomyolysis
aspirin	inhibits thrombus formation	gastric bleeding
streptokinase	acute myocardial infarction	haemorrhage

Further reading

Gibbs, C.R., Davies, M.K., Lip, G.V.H. (2000) *ABC of Heart Failure*. London, BMJ Publishing.
World Health Organization/International Society of Hypertension Guidelines Subcommittee (1993) Guidelines for the management of mild hypertension: memorandum from a WHO/ISH meeting. *J Hypertens* 1993, 11, 905–18.

Website

Cardiovascular drug list:
http://lysine.pharm.utah.edu/netpharm/netpharm_00/dlmaster.htm

CHAPTER 22
Antibiotics

This chapter will cover the general principles of the use of antibiotics in the treatment of infection, with particular emphasis on those antibiotics used in dentistry and the prophylactic use of antibiotics in patients with disorders of the heart valves or prostheses.

Treatment of infection

Antibiotics are among the most commonly used and abused drugs. Several factors need to be taken into account if antibiotics are to be prescribed correctly.

Anatomical location and severity of the infection

Anatomical location gives an idea of the most likely pathogen and suitable drug and determines the route of administration. Infections of the oral cavity most commonly are odontogenic in origin and include dental caries, pulpitis, periapical abscess, gingivitis and periodontal and deep facial space infections.

Although antibiotics given by the oral route are usually enough to achieve adequate tissue concentrations for these infections, intramuscular or intravenous administration will be necessary to achieve these concentrations in life-threatening complications such as intracraneal, retropharyngeal and pleuropulmonary extension and haematogenous dissemination to heart valves, prosthetic devices and other metastatic foci.

Clinical diagnosis of some infective conditions, particularly those of the oral cavity, is sometimes possible since the presentation is typical. However, a diagnosis supported by laboratory confirmation is very important since it allows proper selection of antibiotics. Appropriate specimens should therefore be taken for laboratory investigation before therapy. Knowledge of the local resident flora is very important since it will provide an idea of the possible causative micro-organisms and therefore the choice of the right antimicrobial.

Pre-existing medical problems

Pre-existing medical problems may predispose the patient to infections. These include underlying malignancy, trauma, immuno-suppression, valvular heart disease, prosthetic devices such as heart valves, artificial joints and/or intravascular catheters.

Bactericidal vs bacteriostatic antibiotics

Bactericidal antibiotics kill most bacteria. Bacteriostatic antibiotics only inhibit bacterial growth and therefore rely on host defences to eliminate the infection. If the drug is withdrawn bacteria have the opportunity to recover.

   In the majority of cases the choice between bactericidal or bacteriostatic antibiotics is not critical. The main exceptions are infective endocarditis and neutropenic or immunocompromised patients whose immune response is inappropriate.

Other factors

Drug dosing: Balance should be achieved between toxicity and tolerance.

Length of therapy: This can be assessed clinically but patients should not remain on antibiotics for long periods since complications may arise, such as selection of resistant isolates or adverse reactions. Drug resistance during treatment is uncommon, although some drugs encourage rapid emergence of resistant bacteria. They include: streptomycin, rifampicin, fusidic acid and nalidixic acid. Combined chemotherapy prevents this scenario.

Side effects: Most antibiotics have side effects and these should always be kept in mind.

Cost: Whenever possible it is reasonable to select the cheaper of two equally effective agents.

Failure to respond to treatment

There are many reasons why a patient might not respond to treatment, for example:

• wrong antimicrobial prescribed for the patient's condition.
• inadequate concentration at the site of infection (insufficient dose, inadequate route or poor penetration of the chosen drug).
• presence of necrotic material limits the penetration of the drug, surgical debridement or drainage are necessary for successful outcome.
• infection that occurs in the presence of foreign material such as catheters, prostheses, or any material originating from surgery or trauma will not respond to antibiotic treatment unless the material is removed
• failure to drain an abscess
• lack of compliance.

Prophylaxis of infection

Prophylaxis is the prevention of infection not by immunisation but by administration of antimicrobials. Patients who need this type of prophylaxis are either known to be at risk of a particular infection or are unable to respond to infection because they are immunosuppressed. The main rules for successful prophylaxis with antibiotics are:
• Prophylaxis should be given only at the period of maximum risk so that normal flora is not disturbed and colonisation with resistant micro-organisms does not occur.
• It should be given only to patients in whom the risk of infection is high.
• It should be targeted to specific micro-organisms.
• The agent used should be suitable.
   There are many instances in which prophylaxis with antimicrobials is necessary. It is part of the advice given to travellers in travel clinics, and part of the efforts to control outbreaks. It is used during surgical procedures and in the case of dental procedures it is mostly used for the prevention of infective endocarditis and colonisation/ infection of prostheses.

Infective endocarditis

Infective endocarditis is infection of the endocardial surface of the heart and implies the physical presence of micro-organisms in the lesion. The heart valves are most commonly affected but the disease can also occur on septal defects or on the mural endocardium. The development of infective endocarditis requires the simultaneous occurrence of several independent events:
• Valve surface is altered to produce a suitable site for bacterial attachment and colonisation. These changes may be produced by various local and systemic stresses including blood turbulence.

- Due to the surface changes there is deposition of platelets and fibrin, called non-bacterial thrombotic vegetation (NBTV).
- Bacteria must reach NBTV to adhere and produce colonisation.
- Colonisation once established is covered by fibrin and platelets and this favours bacterial multiplication and vegetation growth.

With pre-existing NBTV, transient bacteraemia may result in colonisation of these lesions. Bacteraemia occurs whenever a mucosal surface heavily colonised with bacteria is traumatised, as in dental extractions and other dental procedures. The degree of bacteraemia is usually proportional to the trauma produced by the procedure and the number of organisms inhabiting the surface. The organisms isolated from the lesions reflect the resident flora of the traumatised area. Patients with a history of rheumatic fever, heart disease with the possibility of valve damage, congenital cardiovascular abnormalities, prosthetic heart valves or arteriosclerosis are subject to deposition of vegetations on the endocardium and therefore should be recognised as high risk and given prophylaxis for dental procedures.

Bactericidal antibiotics are essential for the prophylaxis of infective endocarditis in these conditions. The most common antibiotics used for this purpose are penicillin, amoxicillin and gentamicin. For patients allergic to penicillin, erythromycin, clindamycin or vancomycin should be used. When a patient has been given penicillin or ampicillin in the previous month clindamycin should be used.

Patients who have had infective endocarditis, or who will need general anaesthesia, should be given a dose of ampicillin and gentamicin at induction and one dose of ampicillin or amoxicillin six hours after the procedure. It is important that the agent should be given an hour or so before operation so that peak concentration is present in the blood at the time of maximum risk. Usually one single dose of antibiotic after the procedure is more than enough.

Antibiotics used in dental practice

The most common antibiotics prescribed by dentists for the treatment of dental infections or for use prophylactically, are phenoxymethylpenicillin (Figure 22.1), amoxicillin, erythromycin,

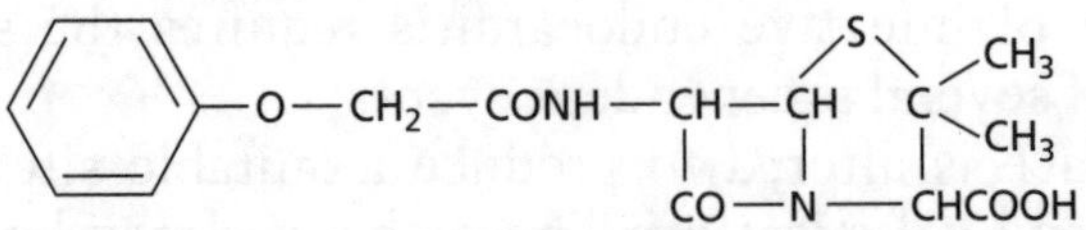

Figure 22.1 The structure of phenoxymethylpenicillin (penicillin V).

Table 22.1 Antibiotics used in dental practice for treatment or prophylaxis

Antibiotic	Type	Site and mode of action	Side effects
penicillin (phenoxymethyl penicillin)	βlactam	cell wall bactericidal	hypersensitivity reactions characterised by anaphylaxis or accelerated/delayed reaction which is less severe seizures with high dosage
amoxycillin	βlactam	cell wall bactericidal	as above non-allergic rash in patients with infectious mononucleosis
erythromycin	macrolide	inhibits protein synthesis bacteriostatic	cholestatic hepatitis could occur
clindamycin	lincosamide	inhibits protein synthesis bacteriostatic	pseudomembranous colitis, since it selects for *Clostridium difficile*
gentamicin	aminoglycoside	inhibits protein synthesis bactericidal	ototoxicity nephrotoxity neuromuscular blockade can reduce respiratory function especially after surgery
metronidazole	nitroimidazole	breakage of DNA bactericidal	reversible peripheral neuropathy with prolonged use avoid alcohol

clindamycin and metronidazole (Table 22.1). The appropriate doses required should be established at the time of prescription by reference to the current edition of a formulary (e.g. the *British National Formulary*, which contains a *Dental Practitioners' Formulary*). Antibiotics may interfere with certain drugs, e.g. warfarin.

Summary: Antibiotics

- **Predisposition to infection** occurs in patients with existing medical problems such as malignancy, trauma, immunosuppression, valvular heart disease, prosthetic heart valves and artificial joints.
- **Failure of an antibiotic** can be due to the wrong drug, inadequate concentration, necrotic tissue or foreign body, or a lack of compliance.
- **Prophylactic use of an antibiotic** should be considered for patients at high risk of infection, for the time of risk, and targeted to specific organisms.
- **Heart patients** are at risk of infective endocarditis if they have thrombotic vegetations on their valves or artificial valves.

Further reading

Lambert, H.P., O'Grady, F., Finch, R., Greenwood, D. (1996) *Antibiotics and Chemotherapy*. 7th edition. Edinburgh, Churchill Livingstone.

Website

Antibiotic prophylaxis guidelines:
http://www.qualitydentistry.com/dental/information/abiotic.html

CHAPTER 23
Immunosuppressants and Corticosteroids

Dentists will rarely be called upon to prescribe corticosteroids and never to prescribe immunosuppressant drugs. However, dealing with a patient already receiving such treatment can certainly worry the dentist and has the potential for harm to the patient. A little background knowledge and some simple practical rules help avoid major pitfalls and should give practising dentists greater confidence. Knowing those diseases commonly treated with immunosuppressant drugs might help identify these patients.

Patient groups treated with immunosuppressant drugs

The largest group of patients treated with immunosuppressant drugs is those with autoimmune diseases such as asthma or rheumatoid arthritis. They are most likely to be treated with corticosteroids, although in some patients alternative immunosuppressant drugs are used to avoid the adverse effects of long-term high-dose corticosteroid use.

In asthma corticosteroids are usually given by inhaler to provide high concentrations in the lung while avoiding adverse effects from absorbed drugs. Patients with malignant disease may receive treatment with cytotoxic drugs that, as an unwanted action, produce immunosuppression. Finally a small group of patients receive immunosuppressant treatment to prevent their bodies rejecting a transplanted organ.

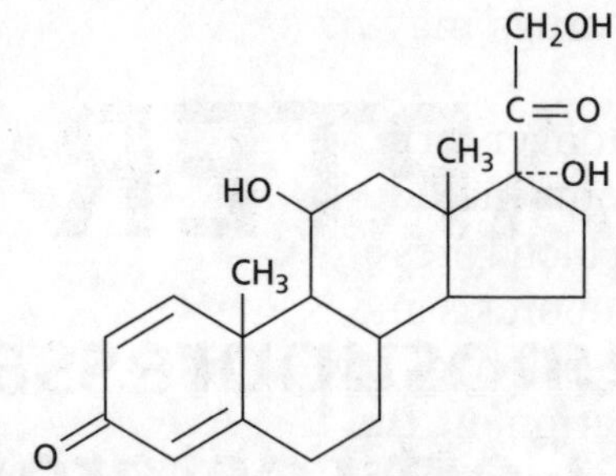

CH₂OH

Figure 23.1 The structure of prednisolone.

Mechanism of action

Immunosuppressant drugs reduce the immune response either by preventing cell division or by interfering with the action of inter-cellular transmitters such as the cytokines. Drugs which interfere with cell division are the common cytotoxic drugs e.g. cyclophosph-amide and chlorambucil or purine/pyrimidine antimetabolites e.g. azathioprine.

Cyclosporin binds to a specific cytoplasmic receptor protein, which limits the phosphorylation of other cytosolic regulatory proteins. In turn, this limits the transcription of several cytokine genes, especially that for interleukin 2. Corticosteroid drugs, e.g. prednisolone (Figure 23.1) have a short-lived effect on the number of circulating lymphocytes probably secondary to redistribution. Their major immunomodulatory action is reducing the transcription of several cytokine genes.

Adverse effects

The immune system is essential in maintaining health by avoiding infection. It is not surprising that suppressing this system increases the risk of infections. These may present either as a more severe form of common and opportunistic infections such as chickenpox or candidiasis (which may affect the mouth), or a disease that does not usually occur in otherwise healthy individuals, such as cytomegalovirus or pneumocystis. Other important adverse effects of immunosuppressant drugs are specific to the class used.

Corticosteroids are fairly well tolerated in the short term although some patients notice sleep disturbance and alteration of mood (high or low). The latter may be marked and precipitate frank psychotic illness. Gingival hypertrophy may be seen with cyclosporin. Some immunosuppressive drugs may be associated with a higher risk of cancer.

In contrast, in the longer term corticosteroids are associated with many different problems including peptic ulceration, fluid retention with consequent high blood pressure or worsening heart failure, induction of diabetes, osteoporosis and proximal myopathy. Of particular importance is suppression of the normal control of endogenous corticosteroid production, at the level of both the adrenal and the pituitary glands. This leaves patients unable to respond to the stress of acute illness or surgery and may persist for some time after corticosteroid drugs are discontinued. For this reason patients treated with corticosteroid drugs should receive specific education about the problem and be instructed to carry a steroid card with them at all times.

Cytotoxic drugs often cause nausea and vomiting, especially immediately after administration, hair loss, and if given during pregnancy damage to the foetus. They can also suppress the production of other bone marrow cells with risk of infection due to lack of neutrophils or bleeding secondary to lack of platelets. The most important adverse effect of cyclosporin is nephrotoxicity, especially important in the renal transplant patient. Hypertension is also common and cyclosporin is one of the many drugs that cause gum hypertrophy and patients with this adverse effect could present initially to their dentist.

Drug interactions

There are surprisingly few drug interactions with immunosuppressants of importance in dentistry. Non-steroidal anti-inflammatory drugs used for pain relief may increase risk of peptic ulceration with corticosteroids and of nephrotoxicity with cyclosporin. Erythromycin and associated antibiotics may inhibit the metabolism of both corticosteroids and cyclosporin increasing the plasma concentration and making toxicity more likely.

Corticosteroids and intercurrent illness/procedures

Patients who present for dental extraction or with dental infection who have received corticosteroids for over three weeks in the preceding year should be given additional corticosteroid on the day of the procedure to achieve a total dose on that day equivalent to prednisolone 10 mg or hydrocortisone 50 mg. Those undergoing major surgery should be given hydrocortisone 50 mg each eight hours for three days. If patients are already receiving greater doses than this then no supplements are required.

Immunosuppressants and corticosteroids in practice

While dentists rarely need to prescribe immunosuppressant drugs, they should be aware of the potential for serious toxicity. The decision to treat should never be taken lightly nor be prescribed by those with little expertise in their use. Before starting treatment with corticosteroids a dentist must decide whether the patient is in a group at high risk of adverse effects, e.g. immune to chickenpox, or postmenopausal women with increased risk of osteoporosis.

Patients need to be given specific warnings about possible adverse effects that might require emergency treatment. These include bone marrow suppression presenting with a throat infection. They should also be told about the need to increase the dose of corticosteroid or even restart such treatment if suffering from an acute illness.

Summary: Immunosuppressants

- **Mechanism of action**: steroids and immunosuppressive agents work by preventing cell division or interfering with cytokine production.
- **Adverse effects**:
  - risk of infection
  - cytotoxic drugs – bone marrow suppression
  - cyclosporin nephrotoxicity – high blood pressure and gum hypertrophy
  - corticosteroids – acute sleep ± mood disturbance, long term – suppression of endogenous steroid production, osteoporosis, peptic ulceration and metabolic effects including raised blood sugar, fluid retention
- **Practical tips**: take advice before prescribing.
- Consider the need for corticosteroid supplements in those usually taking such treatment.

Further reading

Glowniak, J.V., Loriaux, D.L. (1997) A double-blind study of perioperative steroid requirements in secondary adrenal insufficiency. *Surgery* 121, 123–9.

Website

Use of corticosteroids: http://bnf.vhn.net/bnf/documents/bnf.1426.html

CHAPTER 24
Pain: Origins and Control

To manage pain appropriately requires several areas of knowledge to be linked together. In the first instance a diagnosis is required and then appropriate analgesia can be prescribed. Pain is recognised consciously when nerve impulses arrive in the thalamus via the pain pathway. The peripheral receptors for pain are terminal nerve fibres distributed in many organs as a branching network.

Pain fibres enter the spinal cord in the lateral part of the dorsal root. They synapse with neurons that cross to the other side of the spinal cord where they ascend in the lateral spinothalamic tract to the spinal medulla and the thalamus (Figure 24.1). Pain fibres from the face, cornea, tongue, lip and cheek are carried in the trigeminal nerve which enters the brain stem at the pontine region.

Diagnosis

A diagnosis follows from an appropriate history and examination and requires a reasonable level of knowledge of medical conditions that may present with orofacial pain as well as the ability to make a dental diagnosis. Giving appropriate analgesia requires the ability to write a prescription and the knowledge to decide which drugs are appropriate.

Additionally some understanding of simple pharmacokinetics is required to inform decision regarding the route, dose and frequency of administration of the selected drug (Chapter 20, Pharmacokinetics) and a knowledge of side effects and contraindications is important (Chapter 29, Drug Interactions).

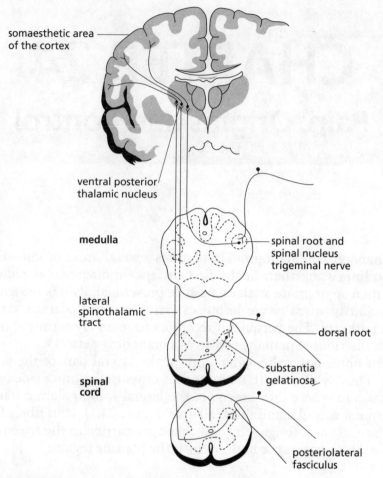

Figure 24.1 The spinal pathways for pain fibres.

Causes of facial pain

Classification of orofacial pain can initially be made according to the anatomical structures present. A reasonable but not exhaustive list would include: teeth, bone, salivary glands, temporomandibular joint (TMJ), sinuses, blood vessels, nerves and skin. Diagnosis will depend upon the ability to take a history and seek clues as to the character, frequency and duration of the pain as well as any physical signs that will point to the specific cause of the pain.

Teeth: The most common cause of pain will be from the teeth and surrounding structures and will usually be associated with caries, although disease of the gingival and mucosal surfaces should also be considered. Mucosal ulcers may be simple aphthous ulcers or may be evidence of viral infection or, rarely, Stevens–Johnson syndrome.

Gross bacterial infection may lead to abscess formation, and impaction of teeth may cause pain.

Bone: Bone pain is typically a result of acute trauma, however, generalised disease of bone may present with facial pain. Both acromegaly and Paget's disease are associated with pain due to expansion of bone tissue. Similarly growth of tumours may cause local pain or pain due to pressure on surrounding tissues.

Salivary glands: The most common salivary gland cause of pain is viral infection in the parotid gland (mumps) but stone formation may occur in the submandibular or parotid glands. Localised tenderness and swelling will usually be present and be exacerbated at meal times.

Temporomandibular joint (TMJ): Pain associated with the TMJ may occur in relation to the articular surface, malocclusion or a muscle disorder. A number of syndromes have been described which can be categorised into internal derangement of the TMJ or pain and dysfunction of myofascial origin.

Sinuses: Sinus pain will usually be due to local infection although tumours may occur.

Blood vessels: Various abnormalities of blood vessels should be considered including temporal arteritis, migraine and cluster headaches.

Nerves: Trigeminal or other forms of neuralgia should be considered, although herpes zoster (shingles) is likely to be the most common cause.

Skin: Local skin infection will usually be self apparent.

The vast majority of patients will have a physical cause for their pain, although this will not always be immediately apparent and may require referral to a specialist. It is also important not to forget causes of pain that may be referred to the orofacial area. Myocardial infarction may present with referred pain to the face or more commonly to the angle of the jaw.

Although psychological problems may present with pain in some individuals, such a diagnosis is primarily one that follows exclusion of possible physical causes.

Analgesia

The choice between the different types of analgesics requires an understanding of their mechanisms of action (Table 24.1) and an

Table 24.1 Site of action and mechanisms of analgesic drugs

Site of action	Drug	Mechanism
tissue/receptor	1. paracetamol, NSAID (e.g. diclofenac)	reduced inflammatory response via cyclo-oxygenase
	2. opioids (e.g. morphine)	activation of peripheral opioid receptors in inflamed tissue
	3. local anaesthetics (local infiltration)	reduced conduction
nerves	local anaesthetics (nerve block)	reduced transmission
spinal cord	1. local anaesthetics	reduced transmission
	2. opioids	opioid receptors in spinal cord modulate transmission
brain	opioids	opioids alter perception of pain

assessment of the severity of the pain. Pain is a subjective response to actual or perceived tissue damage and requires an assessment from the patient and not a judgement by the practitioner. Severe pain is likely to require a more potent analgesic than mild pain and the majority of patients will have already taken simple analgesics such as paracetamol.

Types

Simple analgesics such as paracetamol are used for mild pain. Non-steroidal analgesics (NSAIDs) including ibuprofen and voltarol are often prescribed for moderate pain. Opioids are used in severe pain. Potency varies, with codeine being weaker and morphine stronger. Other drugs may also be used, most often in chronic pain. Antidepressants such as amitriptyline alter central serotonin concentrations. Drugs with combined effects may also be used, e.g. tramadol is an opioid agonist but also affects reuptake of noradrenaline and serotonin release. Co-analgesics are a combination of two drugs, most commonly paracetamol and a varied doses of codeine (8–30 mg) and may be used for moderate pain where a single agent is ineffective.

Administration

Drugs should be given proactively so that they can be absorbed before the severity of pain becomes excessive. This may be as a preoperative dose when surgery is contemplated or when pain 'commences' after a local anaesthetic block, rather than when the pain becomes severe. The route of the analgesic should be appropriate.

Oral route can be used for any drug where absorption from the stomach will take place reliably.

Initial management of severe pain after surgery may require parenteral administration (intramuscular or intravenous) to speed absorption and the onset of analgesia. Parenteral drugs may also be required if absorption is less reliable, such as after major surgery.

Rather than give just a single drug it is also common to use two or more drugs with different modes of activity to increase analgesia without increasing side effects. These effects may be additive or synergistic. For example, paracetamol may be ineffective on its own and a NSAID may improve matters but not remove the pain completely. Yet addition of paracetamol to the NSAID may make the patient pain-free.

Summary: Pain

- **Causes**
  - **Teeth**: caries, abscess, impaction.
  - **Bone**: acromegaly, Paget's disease.
  - **TMJ**: articular – arthritis, extra-articular – malocclusion, muscle spasm.
  - **Salivary glands**: stone, infection.
  - **Sinuses**: infection, tumour.
  - **Blood vessels**: temporal arteritis, migraine, cluster headaches.
  - **Nerves**: trigeminal (or other forms) neuralgia, herpes zoster.
  - **Skin**: local infection.
  - **Psychogenic**.
- **Analgesia**
  - **Mild pain**: simple analgesia, e.g. paracetamol.
  - **Moderate pain**: NSAID, e.g. voltarol.
  - **Severe pain**: opioid, e.g. morphine orally or parenterally.

Further reading

Sharav, Y. Orofacial pain. In: Wall, P.D., Melzack, R. (eds) (1994) *Textbook of Pain*. 3rd edition. Edinburgh, Churchill Livingstone, pp. 563–82.

Website

Postoperative pain:
  http://www.anesthesiology.de/Links/Postoperative_Pain/
  postoperative_pain.htm

CHAPTER 25
Analgesics, Sedatives and Hypnotics

Before painkilling or analgesic drugs can be prescribed safely it is helpful to know a little about how they work and what adverse effects they can cause. The major classes of analgesic drugs in use are the opiates, e.g. morphine or codeine, non-steroidal anti-inflammatory drugs (NSAIDs), e.g. aspirin or ibuprofen, and paracetamol (Figure 25.1).

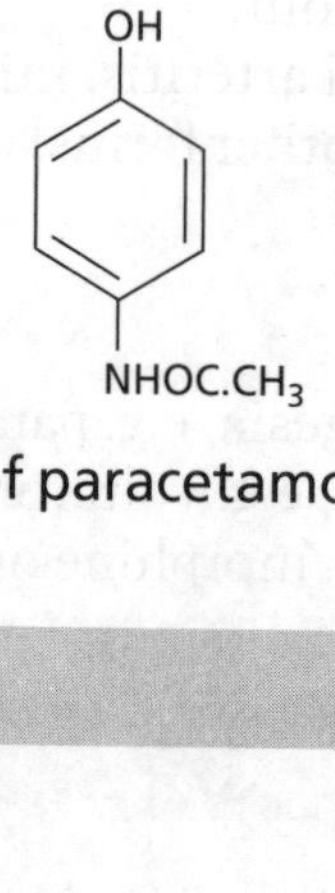

OH

NHOC.CH₃

Figure 25.1 The structure of paracetamol.

Analgesics

Mechanism of action

Each of theses classes has a distinct mechanism of action although that for paracetamol has not been completely elucidated. Opioids bind to specific receptors in the spinal cord and brain that normally modulate the transmission and perception of pain in response to the presence of intrinsic ligands the encephalins and endorphins. NSAIDs inhibit the enzyme cyclo-oxygenase responsible for prostaglandin production.

Prostaglandins themselves do not take part in pain transmission but sensitise peripheral pain receptors, so blocking prostaglandin production diminishes pain perception. Although no one really knows how paracetamol works, the most often quoted story is that it inhibits cyclo-oxygenase in the central nervous system.

Adverse effects

With opioids the most common adverse effects are gastrointestinal problems of nausea, vomiting and constipation. Respiratory depression occurs if such drugs are given, particularly at high dose, but this is usually only a problem when given by injection or in patients with pre-existing chest disease.

Addiction occurs to most if not all opiates but the person most at risk is the prescribing doctor or the nurse giving the injection. Fear of addiction should never inhibit prescribing for pain relief. NSAIDs cause gastrointestinal ulceration, especially in elderly patients who are commonly prescribed these drugs.

NSAIDs vary in their potential to cause gastrointestinal bleeding and ibuprofen is probably the safest drug in this class. Newer NSAIDs are being introduced which have the potential to be safer still. NSAIDs can also cause fluid retention, raised blood pressure and renal impairment. In patients with asthma worsened by aspirin NSAIDs can precipitate an acute attack.

Paracetamol used at therapeutic doses is rarely toxic. In overdose, however, it is very harmful due to a toxic metabolite N-acetyl-β-benzoquinoneimine that although handled effectively following therapeutic doses overwhelms the liver's limited metabolic capacity after an overdose.

Practical use

Most dental pain is of short duration and responds to simple analgesics such as paracetamol or ibuprofen. Occasionally postoperative pain will require an opiate, and morphine given by injection is still useful here. For patients with severe chronic pain, such as that seen with cancer, a stepwise regimen is used starting with simple analgesics then adding weak opioids and eventually strong opioids until relief is achieved. The aim is to pre-empt pain rather than alleviating it once it is felt.

Summary: Analgesics

- **Paracetamol**: useful for minor pain, dangerous only in overdose.
- **NSAIDs**: used for acute pain, avoid in patients with known peptic ulcers or whose asthma is worsened by aspirin.

- **Opioids**: used for severe pain after surgery or chronic pain not responding to simple analgesics. Take care to avoid respiratory depression when administering by injection. Special requirements for writing prescriptions, as these are Controlled Drugs.

Sedatives and hypnotics

Although sedation for an acute procedure, relief from long-term anxiety and induction of sleep are quite distinct aims, the same or similar drugs are often used to achieve all three. The principal aim in one context may be an adverse effect in another e.g. excess drowsiness with an anxiolytic.

The commonest drugs in this class are the benzodiazepines, e.g. diazepam or midazolam, which can be used for all three purposes, while drugs such as zolpidem are used only as hypnotics. The selective $5HT_{1A}$ agonist buspirone can also be used as a hypnotic.

Mechanism of action

The majority of these drugs work by interacting with the receptor for gamma-aminobutyric acid (GABA) in the central nervous system (CNS). GABA is the main inhibitory neurotransmitter in mammals. Although direct GABA agonists have no therapeutic value, drugs that alter the affinity of the receptor for GABA have great utility.

Benzodiazepines bind to part of the GABA receptor that increases its affinity for GABA, while selective GABA receptor binders such as zolpidem and zopiclone bind either to a different region of the GABA receptor or to a limited subset of GABA receptors. The mechanism behind $5HT_{1A}$ agonists induced hypnosis is unknown although it is of interest that unlike the benzodiazepines they do not cause sedation.

Adverse effects

When compared with old sedative drugs like the barbiturates benzodiazepines are extremely safe in routine and even in overdose. When given by mouth they only cause marked CNS depression if given with other drugs such as alcohol. However, midazolam given intravenously can cause severe sedation and respiratory depression, especially if given too rapidly. This is a problem as the sedative action is delayed and it is important to wait to determine the maximum effect before titrating the dose upwards.

Other adverse effects of benzodiazepines are confusion and paradoxical aggression. Originally thought to be non-addictive, benzodiazepines are now known to cause dependence and this is often seen in groups previously not considered at risk of drug abuse. Older formulations of diazepam caused local irritation when injected intravenously. This is not seen with the water-soluble midazolam.

Practical use

In practical use dentists will use injected benzodiazepines in conjunction with local anaesthesia or, less commonly, given by mouth as anxiolytics in patients where the prospect of dental treatment causes severe distress.

Perhaps the commonest drug used intravenously is midazolam and the key practical point is to wait a full two minutes after the initial slow injection to determine response before injecting much smaller increments as required. When used as anxiolytics, benzodiazepines should always be used at the lowest effective dose for as short a time as possible to avoid dependence.

Summary: Sedatives and hypnotics

• **Midazolam** used for intravenous sedation: inject initial dose slowly and then wait two minutes for response before injecting further smaller increments.
• **Benzodiazepines** used as hypnotics or anxiolytics: avoid if possible and use only in short courses. Dependence is possible.

Further reading

Neal, M.J. (2001) *Medical Pharmacology at a Glance*. 4th edition. Oxford, Blackwell Science.
Nutt, D.J. (1990) The pharmacology of human anxiety. *Pharmacology & Therapeutics* 47, 233–66.

Website

Pain relief administered orally:
  http://bnf.vhn.net/bnf/documents/bnf.1426.html

CHAPTER 26
General Anaesthesia

General anaesthesia is no longer given in British general dental practice, but it continues to be an important part of hospital dental work and so dentists need to be familiar with the topic. The aim of this chapter is to give students of dentistry an understanding of anaesthesia for dental procedures. Detailed descriptions of anaesthetic equipment and anaesthetics focus on those used during dental practice.

Locations for general anaesthesia for dental procedures

In the UK, before the 1990 document *'Review of General Anaesthesia and Conscious Sedation in Primary Dental Care'* was issued by the Poswillo committee, general anaesthesia could be performed in a dental practice, providing the recommended criteria were met. However, an analysis of primary dental practices showed that most dentists were not following the guidelines laid down by Poswillo's report. In addition, for at least 70% of those procedures where general anaesthesia was given for simple dental procedures, local anaesthetic would have been adequate.

In the years 1990 to 2000, each year two or three patients, usually children, died under general anaesthesia. In most cases this was due to poor practice (Christie, 2000) and not to unforeseen anaesthetic complications such as anaphylaxis. In 2000, the British government published a report, and general anaesthesia in primary dental practice was banned. This measure will undoubtedly save lives. General anaesthesia at hospitals for dental surgery remains a regular practice.

Anaesthesia for minor dental procedures

Procedures suitable for day case surgery

Minor dental procedures including caries treatment, conservation, multiple extractions, and other dental procedures where the duration of surgery is less than 75 minutes.

Clinical indications: Failure of surgery under local anaesthesia, presence of sepsis making local anaesthetics ineffective, excessive surgical traction required and bone work.

Patient selection: Absolute patient refusal for surgery under local anaesthesia, needle phobia, unco-operative subjects such as the learning disabled. Children are the largest group receiving general anaesthesia for minor dental procedures. Patients should fulfil the local criteria for suitability for day case surgery.
• American Society of Anesthesiologists (ASA) class I (no medical problems) and ASA II (mild medical problems that are controlled)
• responsible adult to escort them home
• residing within a reasonable distance of local hospital
• transport to and from hospital
• telephone at place of residence to contact hospital in case of emergency.

Preoperative assessment: For minor dental procedures the dentist will select and assess cases following local guidelines. Inquiry should be made of a history of previous anaesthesia and a family history of complications following anaesthesia. A past or current history of cardiac disease, respiratory disease, diabetes and neuro-muscular disease should be sought. The assessor should consider if these diseases are stable and controlled or poorly controlled. Contentious cases can be discussed with the local anaesthetic department.

Preoperative investigations (e.g. blood count, ECG and respiratory function tests) are rarely required. A sickle test in at-risk groups is essential. The subject should be given a fasting schedule with their operative date. Should the subject develop a respiratory tract infection before their date of admission they should contact the dental hospital. This will avoid unnecessary cancellations, and a later admission date can be offered.

The anaesthetic: most general anaesthetics for minor dental procedures are administered to children aged between three and eight years. The following description will principally consider children.

Preoperative evaluation includes a thorough history and examination as appropriate. The history should consider recent respiratory tract infections, a history of heart murmurs necessitating the provision of antibiotic prophylaxis, allergies, current medication, a history of general anaesthesia and a family history of anaesthetic complications. Neuromuscular diseases usually preclude the use of suxamethonium.

This will be the first opportunity the anaesthetist has of meeting the patient. They should not feel pressurised into administering an anaesthetic if there is doubt about the safety of the planned procedure. The anaesthetist should take time to explain the procedure to the patient and the parents. The parents are usually given the opportunity to be present during the induction of anaesthesia.

Induction of anaesthesia: Induction is the process whereby the patient is rendered insensible to pain, usually accompanied with loss of consciousness. The theatre environment should be calm. Murals on the walls and ceiling are a useful distraction. The child should be given the opportunity to sit on a parent's knee or sit or lie on the theatre table. Induction may be through the administration of an intravenous agent through an indwelling cannula, or the use of a vapour that the patient inhales through a mask.

For minor dental procedures, of which the majority are carried out in children, the inhalational route is preferred. This avoids the insertion of an indwelling cannula. Of the volatile agents that are available, sevoflurane and halothane are the most satisfactory for the purpose of induction of anaesthesia. The patient, the anaesthetist or the accompanying parent need to hold the facemask so that it covers the mouth and nose, excluding the inhalation of room air. Induction can initially be with nitrous oxide in oxygen and the volatile agent gradually introduced. In the case of a very unco-operative child, high concentrations of a volatile agent are administered at the start.

Maintenance of anaesthesia: Anaesthesia is maintained with a volatile agent, combined with nitrous oxide in oxygen. If sevoflurane or halothane was used for induction these are often used for maintenance, though any of the volatile agents are acceptable.

Airway management: The airway needs to be protected from blood and debris produced during surgery. There is an assumption made that for elective surgery the patient is starved and that there is little likelihood of gastric contents being regurgitated and aspirated. The skilled anaesthetist will maintain anaesthesia with a nasal mask and the jaw thrust manoeuvre. This prevents the tongue falling back against the pharynx and obstructing the airway.

During surgery the surgeon places a pack at the back of the hard palate. This prevents debris falling into the airway and maintains the nasal airway. The anaesthetist will monitor respiration through observation of the capnograph trace and the movements of the bag in the breathing circuit.

Termination of anaesthesia: 100% oxygen is administered, and the patient is turned on their left side.

Analgesia: Paracetamol and a non-steroidal are often sufficient for minor dental procedures. Topical local anaesthesia or infiltration can be a useful adjunct.

Anaesthesia for major dental procedures

Procedures: These include difficult extractions with extensive bone work, third molar extractions, other maxillofacial procedures.

Clinical indications: Patient risk factors where a day case procedure is inappropriate, e.g. cardiac or respiratory disease, progressive neuromuscular diseases, history of general anaesthetic problems, difficult airway, very young children.

Preoperative evaluation: The surgeon is initially responsible for risk assessment, following local guidelines. Referral of difficult cases to the anaesthetic department can be made. If necessary, preoperative admission and assessment are arranged.

Anaesthetic induction: In the UK, anaesthesia is induced in a room adjoining the theatre. An intravenous or inhalational induction may be chosen. Propofol is the intravenous agent of choice: it is a short acting agent with little hangover effect and has an antiemetic effect. Other agents used less commonly include thiopentone, etomidate and ketamine. Sevoflurane or halothane are the inhalational agents of choice. Intravenous access is usually established before induction. Maintenance intravenous fluid is commenced at this time, reducing the risk of postoperative vomiting and the incidence of perioperative hypotension.

Maintenance: The usual choice is maintenance with any of the volatile agents in combination with nitrous oxide and oxygen. Maintenance of anaesthesia with an intravenous propofol infusion is occasionally indicated.

Muscle relaxation: Where intubation and controlled ventilation is used, agents that prevent spontaneous neuromuscular activity are indicated. These are referred to as neuromuscular blocking agents and they all interfere with normal transmission at the neuromuscular junction.

The agents differ in their time of onset, duration of action and side effects. Suxamethonium is unique in its rapid speed of onset and offset of neuromuscular blockade, but the drawback is that it may result in bradycardia or postoperative muscle pain, and it has a high rate of anaphylactic reactions compared with other agents.

In addition, cardiac arrest due to rises in serum potassium of 4.0 mmol is reported in at risk groups. It is used only in the unstarved patient or those who report significant oesophageal reflux where the airway needs to be rapidly secured. Other agents in regular use as neuromuscular blocking agents include mivacurium, vecuronium, atracurium, rocuronium and pancuronium.

Airway: The nature of the surgery or the patient usually excludes spontaneous ventilation with a nasal mask. The options open to the anaesthetist include spontaneous or controlled ventilation with a laryngeal mask. This is managed with a nasal or oral endotracheal tube. Endotracheal intubation involves the passage of a tube, either through the nose or the mouth, and into the upper part of the trachea through the larynx. A laryngoscope facilitates visualisation of the larynx. The endotracheal tube has a cuff at its distal end that, when inflated with air, reduces the risk of solid or liquid from the pharynx soiling the trachea. The anaesthetist uses a pharyngeal gauze pack as a barrier to protect the larynx from soiling.

The laryngeal mask airway (LMA) has two components. The distal part of the LMA conforms to the shape off the pharynx by way of an inflatable cuff and sits above the larynx. The proximal part connects to the anaesthetic breathing circuit. The LMA is placed blindly in the pharynx though the mouth. The disadvantage of the LMA is that it does not prevent the aspiration of regurgitated stomach contents nor blood or foreign material in the mouth.

The surgeon may find his operative field obstructed by the cuffed distal end or the connecting tube. For these reasons the LMA has not found universal popularity for use in dental surgery despite its acceptance in other forms of surgery. The combination of spontaneous ventilation that results in hypercarbia, an endotracheal tube, halothane and infiltration with an adrenaline containing local anaesthetic has in the past produced severe arrhythmias or cardiac arrest and is therefore not to be recommended. The use of sevoflurane and controlled ventilation has reduced this risk considerably.

Recovery and analgesia: Volatile or intravenous agents are stopped at or near the end of the surgical procedure. If a neuromuscular blocking agent has been given, neostigmine in combination with atropine is given. The neostigmine will antagonise the neuromuscular blockade. Spontaneous ventilation is allowed to return. The patient is extubated on their left side with a head down tilt.

Analgesia is provided with a combination of local anaesthetic infiltration, paracetamol, non-steroidal agents and opioids. The degree of postoperative pain suffered by the patient can only be estimated during the procedure. Additional analgesia may need to be administered in the postanaesthetic care unit.

Anaesthesia for the 'special needs' patient

Needle phobic patients have difficulty co-operating with local anaesthesia for dental work. Many other patients with mental and physical problems present a challenge when it comes to administration of an anaesthetic. Patients with learning disabilities, through poor dental care, frequently present for minor dental treatment. Some patients with Down's syndrome, for example, may have difficulty co-operating with dental treatment under local anaesthesia.

Behavioural problems: Some patients may be resistant to coming to hospital and or the theatre. Gentle persuasion, and being accompanied by their immediate carer, may be effective. Alternatively, oral or intramuscular sedation can be used to control disruptive behavior and facilitate treatment.

Pathophysiology: In addition to the learning disability a complex of other physical abnormalities may be present. These include congenital complex cardiac abnormalities, cervical spine instability, facial deformities, large tongue, hydrocephalus, neuromuscular abnormalities and obesity. These may all present specific difficulties for the anaesthetist.

Consent to treatment: The basic elements of informed consent are competency, knowledge and willingness. The special needs patient may, through incapacity or incompetence, be unable to give informed consent to the procedure. The consent, then, needs to be taken from a surrogate decision maker, parent or guardian. Refusal of treatment is common in the special needs patient. Caution should be advised in the use of sedative premedication to facilitate treatment. The clinician should satisfy himself that he is acting in the best interests of the patient, and that there are no conflicts of interest.

Anaesthesia: The special needs patient may have complex patho-physiological problems and be receiving polypharmacy to control behaviour. Adequate preoperative evaluation and investigations may be absent. The anaesthetist needs to balance any risk to the patient against the difficulties of a comprehensive preoperative evaluation. Dental surgical procedures are frequently minor, and so will follow the description for anaesthesia for minor dental procedures described earlier. Patient refusal may, on occasion, require heavy sedation to facilitate treatment. This may include oral midazolam or other benzodiazepines. Intramuscular ketamine is occasionally appropriate in the patient who refuses oral premedication.

Preoperative and postoperative considerations: Patients with special needs require sensitive handling. Their carers need to understand what is involved, why and how to cope with subsequent problems. The ward, theatre and recovery staff need to understand the difficulties and limitations of dealing with these patients, who may not tolerate the normal theatre routine and may prove difficult to entice into hospital. These patients need treatment tailored to their needs, planned by those who are used to dealing with them. They require hospital facilities and staff at hand to deal with any eventuality.

Anaesthetic complications

This is not a comprehensive list, but represents common complications or the most disastrous.

Immediate
- failure to secure the airway
- laryngospasm or bronchospasm
- cardiac arrest and arrhythmias
- anaphylactic or anaphylactoid reactions
- malignant hyperthemia
- aspiration

Intraoperative
- malignant hyperthermia
- bronchospasm
- arrhythmias

- bleeding
- hypotension

Postoperative
- suxamethonium apnoea
- pain
- aspiration
- nausea and vomiting
- airway obstruction

Summary: General anaesthesia

- The largest group of patients who require a general anaesthetic for maxillofacial surgery are children having multiple extractions as day case procedures.
- These procedures present many challenges for the anaesthetist.
- Current clinical practice has made this safe for most patients.
- The future challenge is to eliminate mortality and reduce dependence on general anaesthesia for many procedures.

References

Poswillo, D.E. (1990) *General Anaesthesia, Sedation and Resuscitation in Dentistry*. Report of an Expert Working Party prepared for the Standing Dental Advisory Committee (Poswillo Report). London, Department of Health.

Department of Health (2000) *Conscious Decision:* A review of the use of general anaesthesia and conscious sedation in primary dental care. Report by a group chaired by the Chief Medical Officer and Chief Dental Officer. London, Department of Health.

Christie, B. (2000) Scotland to ban general anaesthesia in dental surgeries. *Br Med J* 320, 598.

Further reading

Gwinnutt, C.L. (1996) *Lecture Notes on Clinical Anaesthesia*. Oxford, Blackwell Science, 1996.

Websites

Conscious Decision report: http://www.doh.gov.uk/pdfs/conscious.pdf
Risk analysis:
    http://www.healthysystem.virginia.edu/internet/anesthesiology

CHAPTER 27
Local Anaesthetics

This chapter will cover the division between 'ester' and 'amide' agents, the signs of toxicity to local anaesthetics, the safe doses of the agents, and the treatment of local anaesthetic toxicity. Techniques of nerve blockade and regional blockade will not be covered.

Why do you need to know everything about local anaesthetics? Because they are the tools of the dental trade used in practically everyone, and you owe it to your patients. Then you will be able to recognise abreactions and failure of action, and if you are unfortunate enough to have a serious incident with a patient, you are equipped to deal with it and the consequences.

Chemical structure and metabolism

All clinically useful local anaesthetics (LAs) are amino-esters or amino-amides.

$$\text{AMIDE: } -NH-C-CH \qquad \text{ESTER: } -C-O-$$

They are metabolised by liver enzymes and pseudocholinesterase in the plasma. LAs prevent conduction of electrical impulses by the membranes of muscle and nerve cells. The typical LA molecule (the structure of lidocaine is shown in Figure 27.1) is a tertiary amine linked to an aromatic system by an intermediate chain, which contains either an amide or ester linkage. The aromatic end is lipophilic and the tertiary amine end is relatively hydrophilic which, being protonated means it is partially positively charged.

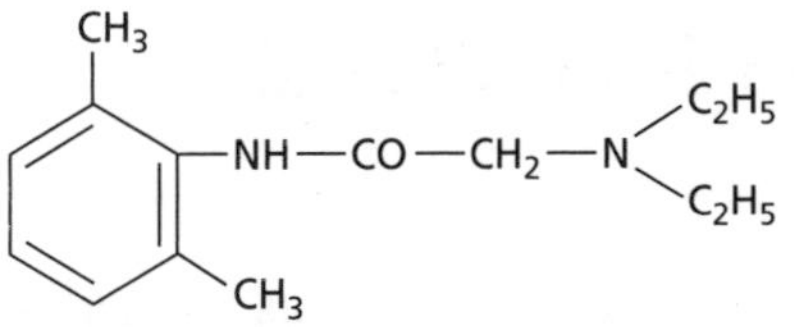

Figure 27.1 The structure of lidocaine (lignocaine).

The relative hydrophobicity and lipophobicity of the LA molecule can be changed by altering the size of either the aromatic end or the tertiary amine end, respectively. The change in nomenclature from –philic to –phobic is due to the bench-testing of these agents in octanol/buffer to test their lipophilicity (known as the partition co-efficient); this was meant to model the drug action in the body. This is satisfactory in the model but no good *in vivo* so the results have been inverted to reflect the physiologically more useful hydrophobicity.

LAs in solution exist in an uncharged basic form (B) and a charged cationic form (BH+). At the pH where 50% of the drug is ionised, and 50% is unionised, the term pK is used. This gives an idea of how ionised the drug is at pH 7.4. The more unionised drug present at the membrane at pH 7.4, the more effective, or potent the agent is, e.g. procaine = pK 8.9; lidocaine (lignocaine) = pK 7.8; and bupivacaine = pK 8.1.

Bupivacaine is more potent than lignocaine – although it is more ionised at pH 7.4, it is 10 times as hydrophobic as lignocaine due to the structure of the aromatic end.

Nerve structure and conduction

In brief, a non-myelinated nerve is an axon wrapped in Schwann cell sheath, a myelinated nerve is an axon wrapped in Schwann plasma membranes. The nodes of Ranvier are important for saltatory conduction. Each nerve axon is wrapped in endoneurium; each bundle of axons is wrapped together as a fasicle, covered in perineurium, and these are bundled together to form the peripheral nerve, and covered with epineurium, which may or may not be myelinated. Therefore the LA diffuses through more than five layers to the site of action.

The nerve resting potential lies at –60 to –90 mV, through the Na+/K+ adenosine triphosphate (ATP)-linked pump that exchanges sodium for potassium. The membranes of the nerve are relatively impermeable to sodium ions and permeable to potassium ions. Ion channels are voltage dependent.

Mechanisms of action of local anaesthetics

Local anaesthetics are manufactured as Cl– salts to aid solubility in plasma. The pH of the tissues and the pKa of the LA agent determines the degree of ionisation in the plasma. The free unionised base diffuses into the neuron, reducing the unionised free base concentration in the surrounding tissues, so more forms from the ionised form in the surrounding tissue. A concentration gradient is set up. This can vary depending on the hydrophobicity of the base and cationic species. Despite the speed of binding to ionic channels, the duration of drug action depends on the diffusion of the LA in and out of the nerve. As the concentration of the local anaesthetic increases, a reduction in the rate and degree of impulse depolarisations is produced. This is not related to the number of Na+ channels blocked.

Clinical pharmacology of local anaesthetics

The potency depends on *in vivo* studies: laboratory results often suggest different rankings to those rankings found in real patients' tissues, (e.g. a LA may be vasodilatory *in vivo*).

The pH of the tissues and the pKa of the LA agent determines the degree of ionisation in the plasma.

Generally the closer the pKa is to the pH, the quicker the onset. However, if a drug (e.g. chloroprocaine) has a pK well adrift, e.g. 9, but is very low toxicity, then LA may be used in much higher concentrations.

• The mass effect of a higher concentration of the same drug causes more rapid onset.

• Very high hydrophobicity may cause much of the drug to get 'trapped' in epineural fat, and not be available to the axon sites.

• Duration of action is chiefly due to intrinsic drug qualities of hydrophobicity but blood wash-out, i.e. drug redistribution is important. Vasoconstrictors prolong block. Low doses of LA have vasoconstrictor activity, high doses, and vasodilation.

• The issue of sensory block (such as in C-fibres) being different, (e.g. in duration) to motor block

• Motor block is not a simple case of size-of-fibres. Vasoconstrictors usually prolong block.

Site of injection matters; peripheral blocks last longer than central (spinal/epidural) blocks.

Table 27.1 Local anaesthetics and their use for infiltration

Group	Local anaesthetic		Without adrenaline		With adrenaline	
	Name	Concentration	Max dose (mg/Kg)	Duration (mins)	Max dose (mg/Kg)	Duration (mins)
Short	procaine chloroprocaine	2%	5–7	15–30	+20%	30–90
Medium	lignocaine	0.5–1%	4.5	30–60	7	120–360
	prilocaine	0.5–1%	8	45–90	+0%	120–360
Long	bupivacaine	0.25–0.5%	1.5–2	120–400	+25%	180–420

Table 27.2 Local anaesthetics and their use for nerve blocks
(dose is as a percentage of infiltration dose)

Group	Local anaesthetic		Without adrenaline		With adrenaline	
	Name	Concentration	Max dose	Duration (mins)	Max dose	Duration (mins)
Short	procaine chloroprocaine	2%	25–50%	15–30	–	30–60
Medium	lignocaine	0.5–1%	50%	30–60	–	120–180
	prilocaine	0.5–1%	25–50%	30–90	–	120–360
Long	bupivacaine	0.25–0.5%	100%	120–400	–	180–420

Practical use of local anaesthetics

Local anaesthetics can be administered by infiltration, topically, intralesionally, intrathecally, as an epidural, spinal, or plexus block. Of the clinically useful LAs, procaine and benzocaine are esters, and lignocaine, prilocaine, bupivacaine (and most others) are amides. Tables 27.1 and 27.2 show the doses and durations of action for infiltration and nerve blocks using LAs.

Pharmacokinetics and toxicity

The concentrations of LAs are higher in better perfused tissues. There is variability between LA drugs in the rate of degradation by liver enzymes and by ester hydrolysis by plasma pseudocholinesterase. The ability to degrade LAs gets less with advancing age. Toxicity is often a variable response depending on rate of absorption from tissue. There is a linear relationship between increasing plasma concentrations and toxic effects. Symptoms include circumoral tingling, lightheadedness, tinnitus, visual disturbance, muscular twitching, convulsion, unconsciousness, respiratory arrest, coma. (The higher the $PaCO_2$, the greater the central nervous system sequestration) and cardiovascular collapse (blocks fast Na+ channels, and Ca++ channels).

Summary: Local anaesthetics

• **Chemical structure**: Local anaesthetics are either amides, e.g. prilocaine, lignocaine and bupivacaine, or esters, e.g. procaine and benzocaine.
• **Mode of action**: LAs work by blocking the impulse depolarisation in nerve fibres.
• **Classification**: LAs can be classified as short-acting, e.g. chloro-procaine, medium-acting, e.g. lignocaine and prilocaine, or long-acting, e.g. bupivacaine.
• **Toxicity** is manifest as circumoral tingling, lightheadedness, convulsion, coma and cardiorespiratory arrest.

Further reading

Malamed, S.F. (1997) *Handbook of Local Anesthesia*. 4th edition. St Louis, Mosby.

Website

Pharmacology of local anaesthetic agents:
    http://www.nda.ox.ac.uk/wfsa/html/u04/u04_014.htm

CHAPTER 28
Maxillofacial Trauma and Anaesthesia

This chapter deals with the management of trauma patients. It emphasises the risks to the patient's airway, the significance of fasting and dehydration, the importance of examining the whole patient and the importance of head injuries and how the airway can be significantly compromised. It is relevant to dentists who may be involved in patients who have sustained trauma to the head and face. The basic principles of resuscitation, i.e. airway, breathing, circulation, apply.

Preoperative assessment

Trauma never occurs as an isolated event to the bit of the face you wish to repair. The patient will have suffered some other injury, or may have been drinking or ingesting intoxicants, or there may be potentially serious legal consequences of the events surrounding the incident.

History

In taking the history of a patient presenting with trauma to the face or head, special attention is paid to the nature and time of the injury, whether there were any witnesses or precipitating factors, and what was the time of last food or drink. Any previous history of collapse, e.g. due to failure of a cardiac pacemaker or alcoholism, should be elicited, along with a drug history, any allergies, a family history of death under anaesthesia, and details of social support (e.g. where does the patient go on discharge?). Questions on the organ systems centre on cardiorespiratory and abdominal symptoms, neurological complaints and the possibility of pregnancy.

Examination

As well as the injury itself, special attention is paid to:
- the patient's mental state
- anaemia
- skin perfusion
- temperature
- jaundice
- bruising
- other injuries
- breathlessness at rest
- an assessment of the cardiovascular state (pulse, blood pressure: is the patient haemorrhaging internally?)
- respiratory function (cyanosis, state of the nasal airways, lung fields, rib fractures)
- abdomen (enlarged liver, injuries)
- nervous system (mental state, cranial nerves, mouth opening, neck movements, limb movements).

If there is any doubt about the patient's mental state, the Glasgow Coma Scale (see Chapter 2, Clinical Examination) should be done, the nurses instructed to undertake neurological observations and probably organise a computerised tomography (CT) head scan.

Investigation

There is a protocol for the investigation of trauma patients based on assessing disease states that present fairly routinely, and based on the broad social factors of age and smoking, guided by the clinical presentation. All patients are investigated by full (complete) blood count and the blood urea, electrolytes and glucose.

Patients over the age of 50 years who are cigarette smokers also have an electrocardiogram (ECG), and those over 60 have an ECG whether they smoke or not. Other tests may include a chest X-ray, skeletal X-rays, a CT head scan, an ultrasound scan of the abdomen, blood tests for clotting, blood cultures, and sometimes echocardiography.

Specific considerations

- Is the patient on any significant drugs (medicinal)?
- Is the patient fasted? (risk of regurgitation and aspiration)

Table 28.1 Clinical features of blood loss

i.e. circulatory volume (for an 80 Kg man, normal pulse 70 bpm, BP 120/80).
The volumes lost do not refer to water loss as in dehydration.

Grade of blood loss	Minimal	Mild	Moderate	Severe
% volume lost	10%	20%	30%	40%
Volume lost	500 ml	1000 ml	1500 ml	2000 ml
Heart rate	normal	100 bpm	120 bpm	140 bpm
Arterial BP (mm Hg)	normal	normal	110/90	60
Mental state	normal	normal	irritable	impaired consciousness
Peripheral circulation	normal	cool/pale	cool/pale + slow capillary refill	cold, clammy, cyanosed
Central venous pressure (mm Hg)	normal	−3	−5	−8

- Has there been blood loss? (see Table 28.1)
- Was there a blow to the head which might produce a subdural or extradural haemorrhage? If so, a CT scan is required before surgery.
- Are there other injuries, e.g. a pneumothorax, and is the cervical spine intact? Can they be moved around in anaesthetised state without damaging the cord?
- Are there other significant medical problems, e.g. drug allergies, HIV or hepatitis risk, illicit drug use, transfusion problems, pregnancy, asthma?
- Who is the next of kin?
- Was the patient involved in an assault?

Rules for general anaesthesia

Patients are never anaesthetised until four hours after drinking clear fluids and six hours after solids. However, because patients who have had facial or head trauma will present technically challenging problems with the management of their airway, an empty stomach is mandatory unless the surgery will be genuinely lifesaving. Passing a nasogastric tube to empty the stomach (lavage) is ineffective and potentially hazardous. The anaesthetist will sort out premedicants and pretreatment such as a blood transfusion and is consulted about any drugs to be prescribed (in case of any drug interactions).

Anaesthetic technique for maxillofacial patients

Dental cases are amongst the most challenging to the anaesthetist, who must induce unconsciousness and maintain respiration without harming the patient. Techniques used for securing the airway include:

• If the patient is fasted, with a straightforward zygoma fracture, and no mouth opening problems then a normal intravenous induction, paralysis, intubation and ventilation anaesthetic are performed.

• If the patient has mouth opening problems due to pain, is suitably fasted and the fracture is undisplaced then unconsciousness is induced without paralysis and laryngoscopy performed to view the larynx. This may include use of a fibre-optic laryngoscope. If it is visible, paralyse, intubate, and ventilate the patient.

• If the patient has gastrointestinal problems, has swallowed a lot of blood, or has difficult fractures with free floating segments, the anaesthetist will do an awake fibre-optic intubation. This takes experience and skilled assistance. If all else fails, emergency tracheostomy may be required.

• The one thing to avoid is the patient losing control of their airway, or breathing, and then finding out that the anatomy of the fractures makes it impossible to ventilate or intubate the patient.

Postoperative management

Postoperatively, the place for recovery must be decided. If the jaws are wired, wire cutters taped to the pillow are mandatory because if the patient vomits and chokes, the consequences are serious. A period of ventilation in the intensive care unit may be required.

Summary: Maxillofacial trauma and anaesthesia

• **Immediate management** of the traumatised patient requires attention to: airway, breathing, circulation, intravenous access, oxygen by mask, sensible intravenous fluid regimen and consideration of analgesia.

• **Preoperative assessment** of the patient with facial trauma include special attention to the nature of the trauma, time of last food or drink, drug history and allergies.

• **Preoperative examination** should include mental state, temperature, cardiovascular readings, respiratory function, neurological state and details of other injuries.

• **Preoperative investigations** should include blood count, blood urea, electrolytes and glucose, and possibly an ECG, chest X-ray, skeletal X-ray or a CT scan of the head.

• **Specific considerations** include whether the patient has taken illicit drugs, is an infective risk, has neck trauma, brain haemorrhage or other injuries.

- **Anaesthetic rules** are that a patient is never anaesthetised within four hours of drinking fluids or six hours of taking solid food.
- **Postoperative management** requires that wire cutters be taped to the pillow if the patient has had their jaw wired. Ventilation in the intensive therapy unit may be required.

Reference

Abrams, K., Grande, C.M. (eds) (1997) *Trauma Anesthesia and Critical Care of Neurological Injury*. New York, Futura Publishing Company.

Website

Emergency medicine: http://erbook.com/

CHAPTER 29
Drug Interactions

The dentist must be aware of the possibility of drug interaction from drugs that he or she may prescribe with any medication that the patient is already taking. Knowledge of the potential consequences of drug interactions may, in some cases, explain symptoms with which a patient may present. The ways in which commonly prescribed and important drugs may interact are shown in Table 29.1. This is not a totally comprehensive list and if the dentist has any doubts, he or she is advised to consult a reference source or the drug information pharmacist at the nearest hospital.

Dentists will see many young women on the **oral contraceptive**. When broad-spectrum antibiotics such as amoxicillin or a tetracycline are given with a combined oestrogen/progestogen pill, there is a possibility of a reduced contraceptive effect.

Local anaesthetics deserve a special mention. Toxicity from a local anaesthetic may occur if it is given in excess or after inadvertent intravascular administration and is manifest as circumoral tingling, lightheadedness, tinnitus, hypotension, bradycardia, visual disturbance, muscular twitching, convulsion, unconsciousness, respiratory arrest and even coma. Hypersensitivity reactions are uncommon with local anaesthetics especially in those of the amide types (i.e. lidocaine, prilocaine, bupivacaine and ropivacaine) but reactions to some preservatives in the local anaesthetics can occur albeit infrequently.

Some drug interactions are possible and are shown in Tables 29.1a and 29.1b.

Table 29.1a Drug interactions for some important and commonly prescribed drugs – overview

	ACE inhibitor	antibiotic	antiepileptic	H2 histamine antagonist	beta blocker	calcium channel blocker	diuretic	non-steroidal	steroid (corticosteroids)	warfarin	local anaesthetics
ACE inhibitor		■		■	■	■	■	■	■		
antibiotic	■		■	■		■	■	■	■	■	■
antiepileptic		■		■	■	■	■	■	■	■	■
H2 histamine antagonist	■	■	■		■	■	■	■		■	■
beta blocker	■		■	■		■	■	■		■	■
calcium channel blocker	■	■	■	■	■		■		■	■	
diuretic	■	■	■	■	■	■		■	■	■	■
non-steroidal	■	■	■	■	■		■			■	■
steroid (corticosteroids)	■	■	■			■	■			■	
warfarin		■	■	■	■	■	■	■	■		
local anaesthetics		■	■	■	■		■	■			

Table 29.1b Drug interactions for some important and commonly prescribed drugs – detail

ACE inhibitor	
antibiotic	tetracycline absorption reduced by quinapril
beta blocker	enhances hypotensive effect
calcium channel blocker	enhances hypotensive effect
diuretic	enhances hypotensive effect
	low plasma K risk
non-steroidal	risk of renal impairment
steroid (corticosteroids)	antagonises hypotensive effect
Antibiotic	
ACE inhibitor	tetracycline absorption reduced by quinapril
antiepileptic	carbamazepine and phenytoin plasma levels may be altered by antibiotics
H2 histamine antagonist	cimetidine may affect plasma levels of some antibiotics
beta blocker	propranolol plasma level decreased by rifampicin
calcium channel blocker	several antibiotics increase or decrease metabolism of CCB
diuretic	loop diuretic increases toxicity of vancomycin and cephalosporin
non-steroidal	NSAIDs give risk of fit with quinolones
steroid (corticosteroids)	erythromycin may inhibit steroid metabolism
warfarin	antibiotics may enhance or reduce anticoagulant effect of warfarin
local anaesthetics	arrhythmias risk with quinupristin, dalfopristin and lidocaine
Antiepileptic	
antibiotic	carbamazepine and phenytoin plasma levels may alter with antibiotics
antiepileptic	two or more antiepileptics may enhance toxicity and side effects
H2 histamine antagonist	cimetidine inhibits antiepileptic metabolism, raising plasma levels
calcium channel blocker	antiepileptic levels can be increased by CCB
	CCB efficacy decreased by phenytoin and carbamazepine
diuretic	risk of low plasma Na with carbamazepine
non-steroidal	NSAIDs may enhance effect of phenytoin
steroid (corticosteroids)	carbamazepine decreases steroid effect
warfarin	carbamazepine enhances metabolism of warfarin
H2 histamine antagonist	
antibiotic	cimetidine may affect plasma levels of some antibiotic
antiepileptic	cimetidine inhibits antiepileptic metabolism, raising plasma levels
H2 histamine antagonist	not normally co-prescribed
beta blocker	cimetidine inhibits beta blocker metabolism, raising plasma levels

Table 29.1b (*cont'd*)

calcium channel blocker	cimetidine inhibits CCB metabolism, raising plasma levels
warfarin	cimetidine enhances anticoagulant effect of warfarin
local anaesthetics	cimetidine inhibits metabolism of lidocaine toxicity risk

Beta blocker

ACE inhibitor	enhances hypotensive effect
antibiotic	propranolol plasma level decreased by rifampicin
H2 histamine antagonist	cimetidine inhibits beta blocker metabolism, raising plasma levels
beta blocker	BBs not normally prescribed together
calcium channel blocker	risk of bradycardia, hypotension and heart failure
diuretic	enhances hypotensive effect
non-steroidal	NSAIDs antagonise hypotensive effect
steroid (corticosteroids)	antagonises hypotensive effect
local anaesthetics	risk of myocardial depression toxicity with propranolol

Calcium channel blocker

ACE inhibitor	enhances hypotensive effect
antibiotic	several antibiotics increase or decrease metabolism of CCBs
antiepileptic	antiepileptic levels can be increased by CCB CCB efficacy decreased by phenytoin and carbamazepine
H2 histamine antagonist	cimetidine inhibits CCB metabolism, raising plasma levels
beta blocker	risk of bradycardia, hypotension and heart failure
calcium channel blocker	CCBs not normally co-prescribed
diuretic	enhances hypotensive effect
steroid (corticosteroids)	antagonises hypotensive effect

Diuretic

ACE inhibitor	enhances hypotensive: low plasma K risk
antibiotic	loop diuretic increases toxicity of vancomycin and cephalosporin
antiepileptic	risk of low plasma Na with carbamazepine
beta blocker	enhances hypotensive effect
calcium channel blocker	enhances hypotensive effect
diuretic	risk of low plasma K and profound diuresis
non-steroidal	risk of renal toxicity risk of increased plasma K with K-sparing diuretics
steroid (corticosteroids)	risk of low plasma K: steroid may antagonise diuretic effect
local anaesthetics	low plasma K from diuretic antagonises effect of lidocaine

Table 29.1b *(cont'd)*

Non-steroidal

ACE inhibitor	risk of renal impairment
antibiotic	risk of fit with quinolones
antiepileptic	may enhance effect of phenytoin
beta blocker	antagonise hypotensive effect
diuretic	risk of renal toxicity, risk of increased plasma K with K-sparing diuretics
non-steroidal	possibly enhances side effects
steroid (corticosteroids)	risk of gastrointestinal bleed and ulceration
warfarin	possibly enhance anticoagulant effect of warfarin

Steroid (corticosteroids)

ACE inhibitor	antagonises hypotensive effect
antibiotic	erythromycin may inhibit steroid metabolism
antiepileptic	carbamazepine decreases steroid effect
beta blocker	antagonises hypotensive effect
calcium channel blocker	antagonises hypotensive effect
diuretic	risk of low plasma K: steroid may antagonise diuretic effect
non-steroidal	risk of gastrointestinal bleed and ulceration
steroid (corticosteroids)	corticosteroids not normally co-prescribed
warfarin	anticoagulant effect of warfarin possibly altered

Warfarin

antibiotic	antibiotics may enhance or reduce anticoagulant effect of warfarin
antiepileptic	carbamazepine enhances metabolism of warfarin
H2 histamine antagonist	cimetidine enhances anticoagulant effect of warfarin
non-steroidal	NSAIDs possibly enhance anticoagulant effect of warfarin
steroid (corticosteroids)	anticoagulant effect of warfarin possibly altered

Local anaesthetics

antibiotic	arrhythmias risk with quinupristin-dalfopristin and lidocaine
H2 histamine antagonist	cimetidine inhibits lidocaine metabolism toxicity risk
beta blocker	risk of myocardial depression: toxicity with propranolol
diuretic	low plasma K from diuretic antagonises effect of lidocaine
local anaesthetics	local anaesthetics not usually co-administered in dental practice

References

Joint Formulary Committee (2003) *British National Formulary*. 45th edition. London, BMJ Publishing.

Stockley, I.H. (1995) *Drug Interactions*. 3rd edition. Oxford, Blackwell Science.

Website

British National Formulary: http://www.bnf.org/

Acknowledgement

The author thanks Mr Richard Glet, Medicines Information Pharmacist, Royal Hallamshire Hospital, Sheffield, England for his kind advice on this section.

SECTION 4
Revision Questions

Problem Solving

Test yourself with these case studies based on material from the book. You should take about 10 minutes to think about and answer each of the questions. Solutions are on pages 255–267.

Cardiovascular disease

1. Chest pain in a patient with a history of cardiac disease

A 60-year-old woman develops tightness in the chest, then chest pain during a routine dental procedure. How should you manage this?

2. Acute shortness of breath

A 72-year-old man develops acute breathlessness, wheezing, anxiety and sweating while waiting to be called in for routine dental treatment. He is bringing up pink frothy sputum, and there are signs of pulmonary oedema. How would you manage this patient?

3. Rigors, night sweats and weight loss in a heart patient

A 57-year-old man presents to your practice for a routine dental check up. On enquiry you find he has had intermittent rigors, night sweats, and weight loss over a period of six weeks. On examination you find him to be anaemic and to have a murmur of aortic incompetence. What diagnosis should you consider? What investigations would help?

Respiratory disease

4. Acute shortness of breath during a procedure

A patient becomes acutely dyspnoeic during a procedure (no previous history). How should you manage this?

5. Home oxygen and dental treatment

A patient who is chronically short of breath and is on home oxygen treatment requires routine dental treatment; what precautions need to be taken?

Gastrointestinal diseases

6. Difficulty swallowing with weight loss

An elderly patient has had difficulty swallowing for the last eight weeks. He has lost weight. What do you need to consider?

7. Retrosternal pain on lying flat

An obese patient develops retrosternal pain radiating to the back on lying flat for dental treatment. What should you consider?

Endocrine diseases and diabetes

8. Increased space between the teeth

A 45-year-old man comes to see you complaining of increasing space between his teeth. What diagnosis should you consider?

9. Dental abscess in a diabetic

A 42-year-old type 1 diabetic patient presents to you with a dental abscess. What is the effect of the dental condition on her diabetes control? How should she manage her diabetes?

10. Aggressive behaviour in a diabetic

Your receptionist reports that your next patient, a 20-year-old man, appears to be confused and is behaving aggressively in the waiting room. You notice from his records that he has insulin-treated diabetes. On investigation you find him sweating profusely and staring into space. What is the cause of his symptoms? What will you do?

Neurological diseases

11. Multiple sclerosis and dental restoration

A patient with relapsing remitting multiple sclerosis needs a dental restoration. What precautions are needed?

12. Seizure (fit) during dental procedure

A patient has a fit during a dental procedure. How should you manage it?

13. Confusion during routine treatment

A patient aged 60 becomes confused during routine dental treatment. What do you need to do?

Renal disease

14. Renal transplant patient needs routine dental treatment

A 58-year-old renal transplant patient who is on conventional immunosuppressive drugs requires routine dental treatment. What precautions would you take?

Haematological disorders

15. Bleeding from an extraction site

A patient who had a single dental extraction returns 48 hours later complaining of continuous oozing from the site of the extraction. How would you investigate him?

16. Dental extraction in a haemophiliac

A patient with known severe haemophilia A requires a dental extraction. What precautions do you need to take?

17. Dental extraction in a patient on warfarin

You need to perform a dental extraction on a patient who takes warfarin because of mitral valve disease and atrial fibrillation. His international normalised ratio (INR) is checked and found to be 3.5, how do you proceed?

18. Bleeding hypertrophic gums with bruising

You examine a patient who came to see you because of bleeding gums. You note that her gums are hypertrophied and that she has bruises on her arms. A year earlier she had major surgery with no complications. How would you investigate her?

Infectious diseases

19. Routine dental care in an HIV positive patient

A patient who is known to be HIV positive requires routine dental treatment. What precautions are needed?

20. Needlestick injury from an HIV positive patient

During a routine dental procedure you sustain a needlestick injury from a patient known to have HIV infection. What action should you take?

Allergy

21. Patient becomes clammy and breathless during routine dental treatment

A 25-year-old woman with a history of atopic eczema undergoes an amalgam restoration and you are wearing latex gloves during the procedure. After 15 minutes, she develops acute swelling of the face and tongue. She becomes pale and clammy with a weak pulse. She feels sick and she cannot breathe properly. It transpires that she neglected to mention that she is allergic to latex. Examination reveals that she feels cool and sweaty. Her pulse is weak. She has a tachycardia. Her blood pressure is unmeasurable. The level of consciousness is falling. Her breathing is laboured.

Ophthalmological disorders

22. Red eyes, dry mouth and facial swelling

A patient with a history of recurrent attacks of acute onset red eyes over the past six months presents with a dry mouth. The patient has been on steroid drops for her eye problems under the supervision of the ophthalmologist. Further questioning reveals a history of swollen parotid glands four months ago, but on examination at present the glands are not swollen. What do you do next?

Dermatological diseases

23. Cheilitis

A patient presents with swelling, cracking and scaling of the lips (cheilitis). The patient has noticed this over the last three or four months but it is not always present and the patient wonders whether the symptoms are related to the use of a specific toothpaste. Examination shows a cheilitis with no changes outside the lips.

24. Intraoral lichenoid eruption

A 50-year-old man, who has been a patient of the practice for more than ten years and has quite heavy amalgam restorations, gives a six-month history of irritation on the buccal mucosa. Examination reveals a lichenoid eruption on both right and left buccal mucosal surfaces adjacent to heavy amalgam restorations.

Rheumatological conditions

25. Neck discomfort in a rheumatoid patient for routine treatment

A 57-year-old man attends for a routine dental appointment. He was involved in a road traffic accident the day before and complains of discomfort in his neck. He has had rheumatoid arthritis for five years, well controlled with methotrexate. How would you approach his neck pain?

26. Mouth ulcers, joint pains and rash

A 45-year-old woman present with oral ulceration. You find out she also has joint pains and a rash. What sort of referral may be required?

27. Dry mouth and rheumatoid arthritis

A 60-year-old woman with seropositive, erosive, nodular rheumatoid arthritis presents to you with increasing dryness and discomfort in the mouth. What further questions would you ask and what treatment would you offer?

Psychiatric disorders

28. Anxiety before dental treatment

Tom is 74 years old. He is late for his appointment with the dentist. He has not seen a dentist for 15 years. He cannot sit still. He is shaking and is sweating profusely. He has a tremor and looks very anxious. What could be causing his anxiety?

29. Mute and unkempt

Sarah is 24 years old. She comes to see her dentist for a routine scale and polish. She is virtually mute, looks dishevelled and is thin. What might be wrong?

Pregnancy

30. Dental abscess in pregnancy

A pregnant woman (8 weeks' gestation) presents with a dental abscess. Discuss your management.

31. Filling replacement in pregnancy

A pregnant woman (12 weeks) presents with toothache and you find a broken filling. Discuss your management.

32. Bleeding gums in pregnancy

A pregnant women (32 weeks) presents with bleeding gums. How would you advise and treat the patient?

Accident and emergency medicine

33. A patient collapses during routine treatment

A 55-year-old man collapses during a dental procedure. How do you assess and manage the situation?

34. Fall with head injury

A patient trips and falls in the dental surgery, banging their head. They now appear to be unconscious. Describe your initial management.

Pharmacology and anaesthetics

35. Aortic valve disease and antibiotic cover

A patient with aortic valve disease who has known penicillin allergy requires an antibiotic to cover routine treatment. What would you choose and what dose would you give?

36. Patient on steroids with an intercurrent illness

A patient is on prednisolone 7.5 mg daily having reduced from 10 mg for control of their pemphigus. They present needing treatment for a dental abscess. Their GP's initial antibiotic treatment has caused severe nausea and diarrhoea.

37. Inadequate postoperative pain control

A fit, young patient has had surgery to remove impacted wisdom teeth and the pain is not controlled by paracetamol. What other analgesic drugs may be used to control postoperative pain and what questions should you ask to avoid predictable side-effects?

Short-answer questions

Test yourself with these short-answer questions based on material from the book. You should take about 10 minutes to think about and answer each of the questions. The answers are on pages 267–270.

38. Describe the clinical features of allergic contact dermatitis on the lips and oral mucosa.

39. What methods can be used to stop bleeding from the gums?

40. List four major causes of renal failure.

41. What emergency measures would you take to treat an anaphylactic reaction in your dental surgery?

42. How can secondary brain injury be measured in a patient who has sustained a head injury?

43. What changes should be foreseen in planning major dental work in a patient with chronic bronchitis and emphysema (COAD)?

44. Describe the normal changes which occur in the dentition during pregnancy.

45. Name one major side effect or toxic effect of each of the following: aspirin, tetracycline, gentamicin, amitriptyline, diazepam.

46. List the sites which require examination in a patient with a neck mass presumed to be malignant in nature.

47. Briefly describe four possible causes of unilateral painless acute loss of vision.

48. Describe very briefly the therapeutic usage of beta blockers and beta$_2$ agonists.

49. A patient in your dental chair suddenly becomes short of breath with a respiratory rate of 25 breaths per minute. Specify three conditions that might have caused the breathlessness. What would be your immediate management for each of these conditions?

50. What is acromegaly? Describe the clinical features of this condition.

51a. Name two medical indications for the use of warfarin therapy.
   b. Describe in simple terms how warfarin works as an anticoagulant.
   c. Discuss the requirements for monitoring during long-term treatment and before dental work.

52. What are the potential consequences for a person who becomes infected with hepatitis B?

53. Name five abnormalities you might find on inspection of the hands and nails. What systemic disorders do these signify?

Multiple choice questions

Multiple-choice questions can be used as a quick method of assessing what has been learnt although they are recognised to have limitations in academic examination. More than one answer may be correct, in some cases all five. Answers are on pages 270–271.

Cardiovascular diseases

54. Central chest pain unrelieved by rest is a result of:

(a) a myocardial infarction
(b) oesophageal reflux
(c) pneumothorax
(d) aortic aneurysm
(e) shingles

55. The following are features of congestive cardiac failure:

(a) breathlessness
(b) tachycardia
(c) raised jugular venous pressure
(d) ankle oedema
(e) central cyanosis

56. Bacterial endocarditis:

(a) does not affect prosthetic heart valves
(b) may follow scaling procedures
(c) in the UK is usually caused by *Streptococcus viridans*
(d) may cause a normochromic normocytic anaemia
(e) usually responds fully to a course of amoxicillin for one week

57. Atrial fibrillation:

(a) is less common in the elderly
(b) is usually associated with symptoms of palpitation in the elderly
(c) can be treated with beta adrenoceptor blockers and calcium channel blockers
(d) is the commonest cause of stroke in the elderly
(e) the thromboemolic risk is reduced by aspirin more than warfarin

Respiratory diseases

58. In acute severe asthma:

(a) the chest is always wheezy
(b) both pulse and respiratory rate are high
(c) sedation may be used to allay anxiety

(d) nebulised salbutamol may cause muscular tremors
(e) high percentage oxygen is needed

59. Sudden onset shortness of breath is classically associated with the following conditions:

(a) asthma
(b) emphysema
(c) pulmonary embolism
(d) pneumothorax
(e) pneumonia

60. The treatment of chronic obstructive airways disease includes:

(a) beta receptor antagonists
(b) atropine-like drugs such as ipratropium
(c) aspirin
(d) inhaled steroids
(e) warfarin

61. Haemoptysis is associated with the following conditions:

(a) lung cancer
(b) pulmonary embolism
(c) sarcoidosis
(d) asbestosis
(e) mesothelioma

Gastrointestinal diseases

62. The following are features of chronic liver disease:

(a) spider naevi
(b) thyrotoxicosis
(c) sclerodactyly
(d) fascites
(e) flexion of the fingers due to Dupuytren's contracture

63. Jaundice:

(a) is always accompanied by dark urine and dark stools
(b) can be caused by bacterial infections as well as viral
(c) is accompanied by pain in cancer of the pancreas

(d) is best examined in natural light
(e) can be associated with excessive bleeding after tooth extraction

---

64. Dysphagia (difficulty swallowing) is a feature of:

(a) lobar pneumonia
(b) carcinoma of the oesophagus
(c) systemic sclerosis
(d) hypothyroidism
(e) atrial fibrillation

Endocrinological diseases

---

65. Thyroid goitre:

(a) is always symmetrical around the midline of the neck
(b) moves upwards on tongue protrusion
(c) can be associated with both overactivity and underactivity of the thyroid gland
(d) is usually associated with difficulty in swallowing
(e) can extend behind the sternum

---

66. A female patient with uncontrolled thyrotoxicosis is likely to have:

(a) increased sweating
(b) heart block
(c) resting tremor
(d) lid retraction
(e) menorrhagia

---

67. Diabetes mellitus may present with:

(a) weight loss
(b) increased thirst
(c) the passing of increased volumes of urine
(d) a sensation of pins and needles in the feet
(e) impotence

---

68. Weight loss is a feature of:

(a) over-treatment with oral steroids
(b) carcinoma of the stomach

(c) active inflammatory bowel disease
(d) hypertension
(e) thyrotoxicosis

Renal diseases

69. Patients on dialysis treatment are at risk of:

(a) infections
(b) malnutrition
(c) bleeding diathesis
(d) all of the above
(e) none of the above

70. Renal transplant patients are at risk of:

(a) opportunistic infections
(b) cancer
(c) lymphomas
(d) peptic ulcers
(e) osteoporosis

Neurological diseases

71. A confusional state may result from:

(a) hypoxia
(b) hyponatraemia
(c) benzodiazepine therapy
(d) hypercalcaemia
(e) hypothyroidism

72. The physical signs of a left lower motor neuron lesion of the seventh cranial nerve include:

(a) sparing of the muscles of the forehead on the same side
(b) an inability to close the left eye
(c) loss of power in the left muscles of mastication
(d) hyperacusis if the nerve to stapedius is involved
(e) decreased sensation over the left maxilla and mandible

73. Clinical features of trigeminal neuralgia:

(a) pain is continuous
(b) it is usually located in only one division of the trigeminal nerve
(c) the patient can describe a precise trigger point
(d) dental extraction can be beneficial
(e) the initial drug of choice is a non-steroidal analgesic

74. Atypical facial pain:

(a) is most common in middle aged women
(b) is relatively common
(c) is usually located in the lower jaw
(d) fluctuates
(e) is only diagnosed after exclusion of other pathologies

Haematological diseases

75. An iron deficiency anaemia:

(a) causes pallor of the mucous membranes
(b) in the UK is rarely due to blood loss
(c) results in red blood cells being much larger than normal
(d) is more common in men than women
(e) usually responds to treatment with oral iron

76. The following may lead to excessive haemorrhage after surgery:

(a) haemophilia
(b) thrombocytopenia
(c) warfarin therapy
(d) steroid therapy
(e) iron deficiency anaemia

77. Warfarin:

(a) warfarin treatment for pulmonary embolus can be interrupted safely for one week when dental treatment is required
(b) causes reduction of clotting factors II, VII, IX and X
(c) can have its effects reversed by protamine sulphate
(d) is monitored using the INR
(e) has a short half life

Infectious diseases

78. The blood of an apparently fit intravenous drug abuser is potentially communicable of:

(a) human immunodeficiency virus
(b) hepatitis E
(c) hepatitis C
(d) *Treponema pallidum*
(e) staphylococcus

79. The following statements regarding HIV/AIDS are correct:

(a) the incidence of AIDS in the UK is now decreasing
(b) the risk of seroconversion following a needlestick injury from an HIV positive patient exceeds 10%
(c) the median time from HIV infection to the development of AIDS is less than five years
(d) zidovudine is of proven value in the treatment of symptomatic HIV positive patients
(e) the median life expectancy following AIDS diagnosis exceeds 12 months

80. Oral involvement is seen in the following bacterial sexually transmitted diseases:

(a) primary syphilis
(b) gonorrhoea
(c) *Chlamydia trachomatis*
(d) bacterial vaginosis
(e) congenital syphilis

Allergic disorders

81. Latex allergy:

(a) is usually due to cell-mediated immunity
(b) can cause fatal anaphylaxis
(c) in a latex-allergic patient, the face may swell after contact with a latex glove
(d) is less common in atopics
(e) latex-allergic patients may complain of food allergies

82. Allergic reactions and dentistry:

(a) allergy to local anaesthetics is common
(b) nickel-allergic patients will react if their dental prosthesis contains chromium
(c) flavourings in a toothpaste can cause cheilitis
(d) contact dermatitis in dentists can be prevented by wearing powder-free latex gloves
(e) latex allergy can be detected by a blood test

83. An acute anaphylactic attack is treated with:

(a) intramuscular adrenaline (epinephrine) injection
(b) an antihistamine tablet
(c) steroids
(d) oxygen supplements
(e) intravenous diazepam

Ophthalmological disorders

84. A painful red eye may be caused by:

(a) treatment with benzodiazepines
(b) acute iritis
(c) occlusion of the middle cerebral artery
(d) acute glaucoma
(e) a vitreous haemorrhage

85. A gradual loss of vision may result from:

(a) cataracts
(b) glaucoma
(c) macular degeneration
(d) iritis
(e) conjunctivitis

Ear, Nose and Throat Diseases

86. The following are causes of neck lumps:

(a) goitre
(b) lymph nodes

(c) cystic hygroma
(d) thyroglossal cyst
(e) subungual naevus

87. A mass within a salivary gland:

(a) is commonest in the submandibular gland
(b) 80% of parotid masses are malignant
(c) 80% of minor salivary gland masses are benign
(d) pleomorphic adenomas of the parotid should be enucleated
(e) surgery on the parotid requires care due to cranial nerve VII

88. Acute sinusitis:

(a) usually affects the maxillary sinus
(b) is associated with bleeding from one side of the nose in over 90% of cases
(c) causes nasal obstruction
(d) responds to antimicrobial drug therapy in most cases
(e) may follow dental treatment

Dermatological diseases

89. The following conditions may cause a skin rash associated with oral ulceration:

(a) pemphigus vulgaris
(b) bullous pemphigoid
(c) lichen planus
(d) psoriasis
(e) systemic lupus erythematosus

90. Erysipelas:

(a) is caused by streptococcal infection
(b) is usually treated with oxytetracycline
(c) may cause chronic lymphoedema of the face
(d) is usually a bilateral problem
(e) is a contraindication to skin surgery

91. Pemphigus:

(a) occurs most frequently in the elderly
(b) typically presents with an itchy rash
(c) is treated with systemic corticosteroids
(d) causes large tense fluid filled blisters
(e) commonly involves the mouth

Rheumatological diseases

92. Rheumatoid arthritis:

(a) is a disease of the elderly
(b) typically causes swelling of the distal interphalangeal joints
(c) causes wasting of the small muscles of the hand
(d) patients are allergic to lignocaine in about 50% cases
(e) causes temporomandibular pain

93. The following conditions can be associated with Sjogren's syndrome:

(a) hypergammaglobulinaemia
(b) rheumatoid arthritis
(c) primary biliary cirrhosis
(d) sarcoidosis
(e) lymphoma

94. The following are true of non-steroidal anti-inflammatory drugs:

(a) they are absolutely contraindicated in asthma
(b) they result in renal failure
(c) they may cause gastrointestinal perforation
(d) they may result in postoperative haemorrhage
(e) they can be used with paracetamol

Psychiatric diseases

95. Hallucinations may appear in the following conditions:

(a) Alzheimer's disease
(b) depression
(c) anxiety

(d) confusional states
(e) mania

96. Tricyclic antidepressants:

(a) are safe in overdose
(b) are safe to use in patients with a recent myocardial infarction
(c) frequently result in a dry mouth
(d) may cause sedation
(e) frequently cause anorexia

Pregnancy

97. The following drugs can be safely used in pregnancy:

(a) tetracycline
(b) ibuprofen
(c) nystatin
(d) lidocaine (lignocaine)
(e) penicillin

98. Which of the following statements about dental treatment in pregnancy are true or false:

(a) a pregnant woman should never be X-rayed
(b) the dose of radiation from a full mouth dental series is 800 times less than the dose of radiation from a chest X-ray
(c) mercury amalgam has been proven to be teratogenic
(d) bleeding from the gums is more common in pregnancy
(e) in the second half of pregnancy, many women become hypertensive if they lie flat on their backs

Accident and Emergency Medicine

99. In cardiopulmonary resuscitation:

(a) chest compressions on an adult should be performed at a rate of 100 per minute
(b) when performing chest compressions on an adult, the sternum should be depressed 4–5 cm
(c) when pupils are fixed and dilated, the resuscitation attempt should be abandoned

(d) a precordial thump is appropriate if the cardiac arrest was witnessed
(e) cardiac arrest is diagnosed by performing an ECG

---

100. In association with extradural haematoma (epidural haematoma):

(a) the patient is likely to have a fractured skull
(b) middle meningeal vessel is the commonest cause
(c) following evacuation, there is minimal brain parenchymal damage
(d) classically, the patient has a lucid interval following initial concussion
(e) is the commonest form of serious head injury

Pharmacology and anaesthetics

---

101. Paracetamol:

(a) is excreted unchanged by the kidney
(b) the maximum recommended daily dose for an adult is 4 g
(c) is antipyretic
(d) inhibits coughing
(e) should not be given to patients allergic to aspirin

---

102. Thiazide diuretics (e.g. bendrofluazide):

(a) are used in the treatment of hypertension
(b) cause a brisk diuresis for about two or three hours after dosing
(c) may cause hypokalaemia
(d) is the intravenous diuretic of choice for pulmonary oedema
(e) may cause gout

---

103. Ampicillin:

(a) is active against certain Gram-positive and Gram-negative organisms
(b) is not inactivated by penicillinases
(c) inhibits bacterial wall synthesis
(d) may cause diarrhoea
(e) is associated with foetal abnormalities when used in pregnancy

104. Recognised side effects of orally administered steroid therapy include:

(a) weight loss
(b) osteoporosis
(c) hyperglycaemia
(d) mental disturbances
(e) immunosuppression

105. The following medical conditions are relative contraindications to day-case anaesthesia:

(a) insulin dependent diabetes mellitus
(b) age greater than 65 years
(c) asthma
(d) myocardial infarction one month previously
(e) aortic aneurysm

SECTION 5
Revision Answers

Problem Solving

Cardiovascular disease

1. Chest pain in a patient with a history of cardiac disease

You suspect angina and stop the procedure if possible. Give the patient sublingual glyceryl trinitrate (GTN). The chest pain should subside within 20 minutes. If this is new onset angina, the patient should be admitted to hospital. If the patient is known to have chronic angina and the pain subsides, inform the general practitioner, as an increase in antianginal treatment or referral to a cardiology clinic may be warranted. If the pain does not settle, suspect a myocardial infarction, give the patient 300 mg of aspirin and admit to hospital immediately for monitoring and fibrinolytic therapy if the diagnosis is confirmed.

2. Acute shortness of breath

The patient has acute heart failure. Initially, sit the patient upright and give high concentration oxygen by mask unless there is coexisting chronic hypercapnia. If available, the correct emergency treatment would be to give intravenous frusemide and consider intravenous diamorphine slowly with an antiemetic. If the attack develops in a dental practice, telephone immediately for the emergency services as the patient needs immediate admission to a medical ward or high dependency unit. An intravenous nitrate infusion will reduce preload. If the patient is in fast atrial fibrillation, they should be loaded with digoxin. Intravenous inotropic agents, e.g. dobutamine and/or dopamine may be of value if there is hypotension.

3. Rigors, night sweats and weight loss in a heart patient

The man in this case had infective endocarditis caused by an alpha haemolytic streptococcus. Blood cultures grew the organism, and echocardiography confirmed aortic incompetence but also showed vegetations on the aortic valve. This man had severe dental caries and had three extractions during the period of antibiotic treatment. He subsequently required aortic valve replacement.

Respiratory disease

4. Acute shortness of breath during a procedure

Check there is no obstruction to the airway. Is the patient wheezing? Is the patient rattly or bubbly? (This suggests acute heart failure). Is there chest pain? Is there cyanosis? Ask about previous illnesses – asthma, chronic bronchitis, long-term oxygen therapy at home, heart problems, angina. If there is no history of chronic bronchitis give 60–100% oxygen by mask. If the patient has chronic bronchitis, particularly if on long-term oxygen at home, give 24–28% oxygen by mask or 1–2 l/min by nasal cannulae, or the flow rate the patient normally uses.

If you hear wheezing give a bronchodilator – salbutamol 8–10 puffs by spacer, terbutaline 8–10 puffs by spacer or salbutamol 5 mg by nebuliser. Repeat after 5–10 minutes if necessary. If a nebuliser is used it is important to continue to give oxygen. In asthmatics use the oxygen to drive the nebuliser. In chronic bronchitics use nasal cannulae. If the patient has anginal pain check if they have their GTN spray or tablets with them and give them a dose. Repeat if necessary. Even if the patient improves it would be advisable to phone for an ambulance, particularly if there has been chest pain.

5. Home oxygen and dental treatment

The diagnosis needs to be established. It is most likely to be chronic obstructive pulmonary disease (COPD). Give the patient their usual bronchodilator drugs 20 minutes before the procedure. If they are on continuous steroids or have received frequent courses (more than four) over the last two years give them steroid cover. Give them oxygen during treatment, using the same flow rate as they use at home – excess oxygen may be dangerous. Treat the patient upright to help minimise dyspnoea during the procedure. Sedation is contraindicated.

Gastrointestinal diseases

6. Difficulty swallowing with weight loss

He has no history of neurological disorders. Oral examination reveals no possible contributing factors. The recent onset of symptoms associated with weight loss in an elderly man raises the suspicion of malignant obstruction and you refer the patient to his general medical practitioner. The patient undergoes gastroscopy and is found to have oesophageal carcinoma.

7. Retrosternal pain on lying flat

Further enquiry reveals that the pain is burning in nature and can be precipitated by lying flat, bending over or after a heavy meal. It is frequently eased by antacids. You suspect this might be gastro-oesophageal reflux and advise him to see his general medical practitioner. He is advised to lose weight during which time his symptoms are controlled with acid suppressants.

Endocrine diseases and diabetes

8. Increased space between the teeth

It is important to consider acromegaly. Ask about any change in his facial appearance, the size of hands, ring size, shoe size and whether he has had any headaches. Examination may show a coarse, large tongue, facial features such as thickening of skin, prominent supraorbital ridges and large frontal sinuses. Referral for a full assessment would be indicated if this diagnosis seemed possible from your examination.

9. Dental abscess in a diabetic

A dental abscess is likely to activate the metabolic response to stress. This causes reduced insulin sensitivity (due to an increased production of counter regulatory hormones such as cortisol and catecholamines) and reduced insulin secretion secondary to increased sympathetic activity. Increased catabolism leads to hyperglycaemia, and ketosis.

Your patient should increase her frequency of blood sugar monitoring to at least four times per day and check her urine for ketones. If her blood sugar levels are raised or she has ketonuria she should take her usual dose of quick-acting insulin. If she has difficulty eating she should not reduce or omit any insulin, but should substitute sugary drinks for meals. If she is in doubt about insulin dose adjustments she should liaise with her diabetes team.

10. Aggressive behaviour in a diabetic

Behavioural change is a common presenting symptom of hypoglycaemia. Many patients do not recognise early warning symptoms of hypoglycaemia such as sweating, palpitation or trembling. Their blood sugars continue to drop and neuroglycopenia ensues. In this circumstance patients may exhibit inappropriate behaviour or appear vague. They may refuse sugar and deny hypoglycaemia. This patient is conscious and may be treated with oral carbohydrate. Give a quick acting carbohydrate such as a can of fizzy (non diet) drink, or glucose tablets. Then give some slower acting carbohydrate – such as two digestive biscuits or a packet of crisps – to avoid further hypoglycaemia.

Neurological diseases

11. Multiple sclerosis and dental restoration

No special precautions are needed. Dental treatment, trauma and other exogenous life events influence neither the disease nor its clinical course. Amalgam fillings are not detrimental in any way.

Some investigators claimed that new episodes of demyelination increase after viral exposure (but no single agent has been implicated), and that 9% of infections are followed by relapses.

12. Seizure (fit) during dental procedure

Most seizures self terminate. Usually no treatment is required. Ensure that patient's airways are protected by putting them in the recovery position. Status epilepticus is defined as two or more seizures in succession without recovery in between, or seizure lasting longer than 30 minutes. This is a medical emergency requiring immediate hospital admission and treatment.

13. Confusion during routine treatment

Any physical disease could induce confusion. Stop the procedure and consider the possible causes:

- drugs (especially analgesics and sedatives)
- metabolic disorder (electrolyte imbalance, hypo- and hyperglycaemia)
- hypoxia (particularly in patients with chronic airway disease)
- vascular (stroke, myocardial infarction, pulmonary embolism)
- infection (dental, chest, urinary tract)

Consider further investigations and treatment depending on the suspected cause.

Renal disease

14. Renal transplant patient needs routine dental treatment

Enquire about the patient's renal function. If normal proceed as planned. If abnormal, check bleeding time in case of procedure associated with bleeding. Ask if the patient is on cyclosporin as he may have severe gingival hypertrophy. Listen or enquire about presence/absence of a heart murmur – if absent proceed as planned. If present, give prophylactic antibiotics as recommended by the Working Party of the British Society of Antimicrobial Chemotherapy.

Haematological disorders

15. Bleeding from an extraction site

Suspect a bleeding disorder and take a careful history, asking about easy bruising/bleeding, nosebleeds, bleeding after surgery/trauma/previous dental extractions as well as a family history. Initial investigations should include a full blood count and a clotting screen (which includes a prothrombin time, activated partial thromboplastin time (APTT) and fibrinogen). Although these would be sufficient to identify important causes such as thrombocytopenia and haemophilia, if the results are normal not all important disorders are excluded e.g. platelet function defects. Consider referring the patient to a haematologist for further investigation.

16. Dental extraction in a haemophiliac

This patient will undoubtedly bleed excessively if his extraction is not appropriately managed. Discuss the case with a haematologist. Before the extraction the patient will receive Factor VIII concentrate intravenously to correct the bleeding diathesis. Usually only a single injection is sufficient. Post extraction he should be given tranexamic acid, an antifibrinolytic drug, as a mouthwash to take for five to seven days. If there is any evidence of infection he should be prescribed antibiotics. Intramuscular injections must be avoided as should aspirin and non-steroidal anti-inflammatory drugs. These inhibit platelet function and may worsen the coagulopathy.

17. Dental extraction in a patient on warfarin

Patients with atrial fibrillation are frequently on warfarin to prevent arterial thromboses such as stroke. Warfarin is monitored using the INR test and this patient's ideal INR should have been 2.0–3.0. Any patient on warfarin should have their INR checked on the day of any invasive procedure and you should not rely on their last result. Dental extractions can be carried out provided the INR is less than 3.0.

If the result is higher than this, discuss it with the patient's anti-coagulant clinic who will advise on warfarin dose reduction/omission to get the INR to the desired range. The patients can restart their warfarin on the evening of the dental extraction day. Because of the abnormal mitral valve this patient should receive antibiotics for prophylaxis against subacute bacterial endocarditis.

18. Bleeding hypertrophic gums with bruising

The bruises on her arms and the gum bleeding suggest a coagulation abnormality which must be of recent onset as she had surgery without excessive bleeding. Gum hypertrophy is a feature of acute monocytic leukaemia (as well as drug treatment with phenytoin or cyclosporin). Strongly suspect the diagnosis of acute leukaemia – the bleeding and bruising being due to thrombocytopenia. General bone marrow failure may be present and you should ask about features of anaemia, excessive infections and other bleeding. The most important investigations to request are a full blood count and a coagulation screen.

Infectious diseases

19. Routine dental care in an HIV positive patient

Risks to the dentist in treating HIV positive patients are extremely low. However, you should observe precautions (Department of Health website) to minimise any possible risk of exposure to blood and saliva.
• Do not re-sheath needles.
• Use a neutral area such as a kidney bowl to avoid hand passing sharp instruments from one person to another.

- Ensure sharps are not left in the operative field.
- Remove needles from syringes only when essential – dispose of the whole unit.
- Use instrument rather than fingers for retraction/suturing.
- Double gloving does not prevent percutaneous injury but may reduce the volume inoculated by the wiping effect.
- Reglove as soon as possible if a glove puncture is suspected.
- Wear protective eyewear and mask or face shield.
- Use disposable equipment where possible.
- Dispose of contaminated materials appropriately and ensure all equipment is sterilised after use.

20. Needlestick injury from an HIV positive patient

Wash the injury (do not suck it) and encourage it to bleed. Report the incident to occupational health and seek advice about postexposure prophylaxis (PEP) with antiretroviral drugs. This is recommended for healthcare workers sustaining a significant contamination injury. You should preferably start PEP within one hour of the injury. Arrange HIV testing at an appropriate time (three months) following the injury. The risk of acquiring HIV infection following a needlestick injury from a known HIV positive person is low – 3 per 1000 cases. (Department of Health, www.doh.gov.uk/pub/docs/doh/chcguid1.pdf page 7)

Allergy

21. Patient becomes clammy and breathless during routine dental treatment

You diagnose the problem as acute anaphylactic reaction to latex. You secure her airway, lie her flat and raise her feet, administer oxygen via a facial mask. You inject adrenaline (epinephrine) intramuscularly in a dose of 1 mg (this is 1 ml of an adrenaline injection 1 in 1000). Pulse and blood pressure are monitored. You instruct a member of your staff to telephone 999 for an urgent ambulance, as the patient will need to be taken urgently to an Accident & Emergency Department.

Ophthalmological disorders

22. Red eyes, dry mouth and facial swelling

You suspect that an underlying systemic condition may have caused the red eye, dry mouth and history of swollen parotids. You contact the patient's ophthalmologist to highlight the new complaints of dry mouth. Further investigations are arranged, including chest X-ray and blood tests. The chest X-ray shows hilar lymphadenopathy and blood tests reveal a raised serum ACE (angiotensin converting enzyme).

The diagnosis of sarcoidosis is considered and confirmed by transbronchial lung biopsy which shows typical non-caseating granulomas. Systemic steroids are discussed, but as the disease often resolves on its own, and the patient expresses a strong desire to avoid systemic steroids, this is not used. Local treatment for the eye and symptomatic relief for the dry mouth are provided.

Dermatological diseases

23. Cheilitis

You suspect that this might be an allergic contact dermatitis and refer the patient to her general medical practitioner who arranges an appointment with a dermatologist. Patch testing demonstrates sensitivity to cinnamaldehyde which is identified as a component of the offending toothpaste. Avoidance of this chemical is possible, as products are ingredient labelled, and results in a cure.

24. Intraoral lichenoid eruption

You suspect this may be a hypersensitivity to mercury and refer the patient to the oral medicine clinic at your local dental hospital. There, a biopsy demonstrates a lichenoid eruption. The patient is referred for patch testing which demonstrates contact sensitivity to mercury. The offending large restorations are removed and replaced by composite. Within a few weeks the lichenoid eruption clears.

Rheumatological conditions

25. Neck discomfort in a rheumatoid patient for routine treatment

It is likely that this man had a whiplash injury resulting in soft tissue pain. Rheumatoid subluxation of the cervical spine is unlikely because of the relatively short disease duration and the good control of the disease. It cannot, however, be excluded clinically. The patient should have a full neurological assessment and X-ray of the cervical spine in flexion and extension. Treatment for whiplash is with physiotherapy and analgesics.

26. Mouth ulcers, joint pains and rash

A connective tissue disease may cause these clinical features. Referral to a dermatologist or rheumatologist would be appropriate. The extent and distribution of the rash may define whether the patient has lupus erythematosus, e.g. butterfly rash, the facial erythema and erythematous changes on the extensor aspects of the limbs as in dermatomyositis, or vasculitis as in polyarthritis nodosa.

The distribution and severity of the joint inflammation may differentiate between an inflammatory, symmetrical polyarthritis, as seen in rheumatoid arthritis, or arthralgias or low grade synovitis seen in the connective tissue disorders.

The history of mouth ulcers and examination will reveal whether the ulcers are shallow or deep, painful or painless, the distribution within the mouth, or deep at the back of the pharynx or associated with other more destructive lesions of the nasal passages, sinuses or orbit.

27. Dry mouth and rheumatoid arthritis

A patient with severe rheumatoid arthritis may have secondary Sjogren's syndrome causing dry mouth and dry eyes due to impaired salivary gland and lacrimal gland secretion. The salivary glands may be inflamed, tender and palpably enlarged. Advise the patient about dental hygiene, the importance of keeping the teeth and gums healthy, the importance of visiting the dental hygienist on a regular basis and avoiding smoking. The saliva production may be improved by using sugar-free lozenges to stimulate the secretion and in severe cases artificial saliva may be necessary. Also ask about drugs with a powerful anticholinergic effect, which may aggravate dryness of the mouth.

Psychiatric disorders

28. Anxiety prior to dental treatment

Always think of other causes in psychiatry apart from the most obvious ones. The list of disorders described in Table A1 can provide a basis for building up a differential diagnosis. Tom tells you that he

Table A1 Possible diagnosis and reasons for anxiety before dental treatment

Possible diagnosis	Reasons for diagnosis
Dementia	Anxiety and changes in behaviour can be an early sign of dementia. He is elderly. He has not been to the dentist in 15 years. Could he have forgotten?
Delirium	Confused patients may present with anxiety.
Substance misuse	Withdrawal from alcohol or benzodiazepines.
Schizophrenia	Frightening delusions or hallucinations.
Depression	Anxiety is commonly another feature.
Anxiety disorders	Could have anxiety all the time or it could have been precipitated by the proximity to the dental surgery. Has not been in 15 years. Dental phobia?

Table A2 Possible diagnosis and reasons for being mute and unkempt

Possible diagnosis	Reasons for diagnosis
Substance misuse	Dependence on alcohol or heroin may present with loss of weight and lack of self-care. Depression can be secondary to these disorders.
Schizophrenia	The positive symptoms can be so overwhelming that the sufferer cannot concentrate on everyday life. The negative symptoms create apathy and lack of motivation.
Depression	Patients can lose weight and become despondent. Mutism is a sign of severe depression.

is ashamed but he states that has been frightened of coming to the dentist for 15 years. Tom has dental phobia. The treatment of choice is graded exposure.

29. Mute and unkempt

You consider a number of possible psychiatric diagnoses, as listed in Table A2. Sarah tells you she feels depressed. You notice pinpoint pupils and suspect heroin dependence causing depression.

Pregnancy

30. Dental abscess in pregnancy

Drain the abscess and dress the tooth. Prescribe antibiotics if there is evidence of systemic upset. Defer root canal treatment or extraction until the second trimester.

31. Filling replacement in pregnancy

Under local anaesthesia remove the remains of the old filling and any caries. Stabilise the tooth. Either administer a new filling or extirpate the pulp and place a temporary dressing if exposed. (An X-ray is not essential). If further treatment is needed (i.e. root canal work or extraction) then defer this until the second trimester.

32. Bleeding gums in pregnancy

Scale and polish teeth and reassure your patient that there is no disease present (this is a short appointment of less than 20 minutes). Explain that the changes in the oral cavity in pregnancy predispose to bleeding gums. Advise on oral hygiene to minimise the problem. Encourage home care with a chlorhexidine mouthwash if needed. Arrange a follow-up appointment three months after delivery.

Accident and emergency medicine

33. A patient collapses during routine treatment

You assess the situation for hazards, carefully removing any sharps or equipment. While manoeuvring the dental chair into a horizontal position assess the patient for responsiveness and shout for help. Look in the airway, checking for obstruction and perform suction if necessary, then open the airway with head tilt/chin lift. Check for breathing by looking, listening and feeling for 10 seconds. If your patient is not breathing send someone to dial 999.

Using a protective airway adjunct deliver two effective ventilations then assess the circulation for 10 seconds (carotid pulse/skin colour/movement). If there is no circulation present instruct a colleague to commence chest compressions at a ratio of five compressions to one ventilation. Continue resuscitation until the patient shows signs of life or until the paramedics arrive. Instruct one member of staff to locate the resuscitation equipment kept by your practice and another to wait outside for the ambulance.

34. Fall with head injury

The first aim is to check the ABC status of the patient.

Airway: Inspect the mouth for blood, loose dentures or teeth and vomit. If present, clear any debris by a finger sweep inside the mouth, or by using a suction machine, if portable to the patient.

Do not move the patient. Then recheck the airway. Clear any further debris then use a jaw thrust manoeuvre to keep the airway open.

Breathing: Check for breathing adequacy by looking for the rise and fall of the chest, listening for breath sounds at the mouth and feeling for expired air against your cheek held to the patient's mouth. If breathing is erratic, or fewer than eight breaths per minute, begin assisted ventilation using a pocket mask or bag valve mask device connected to an oxygen supply. If there is no equipment, use a mouth-to-mouth technique. If breathing appears adequate apply an oxygen mask to the patient if available.

Circulation: Check the carotid pulse and if not palpable in an unconscious patient begin cardiopulmonary resuscitation (CPR). If there is a pulse, CPR is not immediately required.

The next aim is to minimise the effects of the head injury. If there are any obvious bleeding scalp or facial wounds apply direct manual pressure using gauze swabs. Cover the patient with a warm blanket or clothing. Unconscious patients, especially the elderly and children, get cold quickly and this hampers recovery. Ensure that someone has called an ambulance and told the control room that you are dealing with an unconscious patient. Make sure the person nominated to call 999 comes back to confirm they have done so. Keep a note of all that you have done as this will assist the people who receive the patient on arrival at A & E.

Pharmacology and anaesthetics

35. Aortic valve disease and antibiotic cover

A patient with aortic valve disease is at risk of developing infective endocarditis. The antibiotic choice in this case is difficult since the patient is allergic to penicillin. Under **local or no** anaesthesia, clindamycin 600 mg one hour before the procedure for adults, 300 mg for 5–10-year-olds and 150 mg for children under 5 years of age, would be the drug of choice.

Under **general** anaesthesia, intravenous vancomycin 1 gram over at least 100 minutes and intravenous gentamicin 120 mg at induction. Intravenous teicoplanin 400 mg can be given instead of vancomycin at induction. Clindamycin intravenous 300 mg over at least 10 minutes at induction and 150 mg oral or intravenous six hours later would also be suitable.

36. Patient on steroids with an intercurrent illness

The patient needs their treatment increasing for the duration of acute illness. As they are probably not absorbing prednisolone because of the vomiting it would be better to give hydrocortisone intravenously.

37. Inadequate postoperative pain control

Local anaesthesia could have been injected at surgery and a minor opioid or a non-steroidal analgesic could now be prescribed, either singly or together if one alone is still not effective. Examples would be bupivacaine, dihydrocodeine and diclofenac. To avoid predictable side effects ask the patient about drug allergies and – because of the NSAID – about a history of peptic ulceration or asthma. If either of these symptoms is present, warn the patient about a possible exacerbation of symptoms due to the NSAID but do not necessarily contraindicate its use.

Websites

British Society for Antimicrobial Chemotherapy:
   http://www.bsac.org.uk/
Expert Advisory Group on AIDS (HIV precautions):
   http://www.doh.gov.uk/eaga/keepsafe1.htm

Short answer questions

Here are what your answers to the questions on pages 239–240 should include:
38. Descriptions of:
- swelling
- redness
- scaling
- blistering
- cracking (fissuring)
- exudation (weeping)
- lichenoid reaction.

39. Establish the cause of bleeding from the history and examination. Treatment may include:
- compression
- suturing
- vitamin K (for over-coagulation with warfarin)
- platelet infusion (for low platelet count)

- fresh frozen plasma (for bleeding due to liver disease or acute treatment for warfarin over-coagulation)
- factor VIII concentrate (for bleeding in a haemophiliac)

Only the first two treatments are likely to be given in the dental practice – emergency services should be called if bleeding is obviously not going to stop.

40. Any four of the following:
- hypertension
- diabetes
- connective tissue disorder
- drug-induced obstructive uropathy
- polycystic kidney disease
- glomerulonephritis

41. In this order:
- ask a member of staff to telephone for the emergency services
- Airways (check that they are clear)
- Breathing (check the patient is breathing)
- Circulation (check pulse and blood pressure).

Secondary measures might include giving adrenaline (subcutaneously or intramuscularly) and oxygen.

42. Can they:
- open their eyes?
- speak?
- comprehend?
- move all limbs?

These assess the level of consciousness. Also note pupil reactions. Mention of the Glasgow Coma Scale would be an excellent answer.

43. The dentist should be aware of the:
- possibility of cyanosis
- correct positioning of the patient (upright)
- need for oxygen supplementation
- possibilities of complications from concurrent steroid administration
- type of postoperative analgesia required
- need for inhaler use if wheezing develops.

44. Pregnancy does not cause gingivitis and bleeding gums are likely. The pregnancy response is associated with an exaggerated production of inflammatory tissue in response to the slightest irritation. This may be mild, e.g. the interdental papillae are swollen and red, or severe where the gingivae are enlarged and plum-coloured. Gingival tumefactions affect about 1% of pregnant women and may be small – an enlarged interdental papilla or occasionally larger (>1 cm diameter).

Gingivitis may be confused with pyogenic granuloma. Removal of gingival tumefactions is often followed by recurrence, so such lesions should be treated after delivery.

Pregnancy may be associated with excessive salivation of unknown cause. Tooth mobility may occur.

45. Side effects or toxic effects
- **aspirin** (bleeding, tinnitus, bronchiospasm, metabolic acidosis)
- **tetracycline** (photosensitivity, gastrointestinal upset, yellowing of teeth)
- **gentamicin** (inner ear damage, renal impairment)
- **amitriptyline** (dry mouth, urinary retention, constipation, blurred vision, cardiac arrhythmia)
- **diazepam** (drowsiness and respiratory depression).

46. Sites to examine include: (any five of the following):
- thyroid
- submandibular, submental or parotid salivary glands
- neck or axilla for lymphadenopathy
- oral cavity
- pharynx
- postnasal space
- (possibly) scalp, chest and breasts.

47. Possible causes include (four of the following):
- embolic phenomenon
- retinal detachment
- vitreous detachment
- retinal artery or retinal vein occlusion
- bleed into the vitreous.

48. Therapeutic use:
- beta blockers are used for angina, hypertension, migraine and for treating anxiety
- $beta_2$ agonists are used for the treatment of asthma and chronic bronchitis

49. Your answer should include three of the following four causes, together with their solutions:
- pulmonary embolism (call help first, check pulse and blood pressure, check airway, give oxygen)
- acute myocardial infarction (as for pulmonary embolism)
- exacerbation of asthma (administer inhalers and oxygen)
- allergic reaction (call help first, attention to airways, breathing and circulation).

50. Acromegaly represents the production of excessive amounts of growth hormone by an anterior pituitary adenoma. Clinical features include:
- spade hands
- prominent jaw
- bitemporal hemianopia
- hypertrophic frontal sinus

- large tongue
- widening of dentition.

51a. Any two of
- atrial fibrillation
- deep vein thrombosis
- pulmonary embolism
- prosthetic heart valve.

51b. The single answer is that warfarin works by blocking the production of vitamin K clotting factors.

51c. The INR of the prothrombin time is estimated. Dental work can be undertaken with an INR of 3.0.

52. Potential consequences of hepatitis B include:
- carrier who may infect others
- chronic hepatitis
- liver cirrhosis
- carcinoma of liver
- liver failure.

53. Abnormalities of hands and nails (and the systemic disorders they signify) include:
- clubbing of nails (indicating heart disease, lung disease, malignancy)
- koilonychia (iron deficiency)
- splinter haemorrhage (infective endocarditis)
- pitting of nails or onycholysis (psoriasis)
- nail fold telangiectasia (connective tissue diseases)
- palmar erythema (liver disease)
- pigmentation of creases (Addison's disease)
- vitiligo (autoimmune disorders)
- pallor (anaemia)
- Dupuytren's contracture (liver disease)
- joint changes (rheumatoid arthritis or of systemic sclerosis)
- spade-like hands (acromegaly, eruption of dermatomyositis).

Multiple choice answers

These are the answers to the multiple choice questions on pages 240–252.

54. (a) (b) (d)
55. all of them
56. (b) (c) (d)
57. (c) (d)
58. (b) (d) (e)
59. (a) (c) (d)
60. (b) (d)

61. (a) (b)
62. (a) (d) (e)
63. (b) (d) (e)
64. (b) (c)
65. (c) (e)
66. (a) (c) (d)
67. all of them
68. (b) (c) (e)
69. (d)
70. (a) (b) (c) (e)
71. all of them
72. (b) (d)
73. (b) (c)
74. (a) (b) (e)
75. (a) (e)
76. (a) (b) (c)
77. (b) (d)
78. (a) (c)
79. (d) (e)
80. (a) (b) (e)
81. (b) (c) (e)
82. (c) (e)
83. (a) (c) (d)
84. (b) (d)
85. (a) (b) (c)
86. (a) (b) (c) (d)
87. (e)
88. (a) (d) (e)
89. (a) (b) (c) (e)
90. (a) (c) (e)
91. (c) (e)
92. (c) (e)
93. all of them
94. all of them
95. (a) (b) (d) (e)
96. (c) (d)
97. (c) (d) (e)
98. (b) (d)
99. (a) (b) (d)
100. (a) (b) (c) (d)
101. (b) (c)
102. (a) (c) (e)
103. (a) (c) (d)
104. (b) (c) (d) (e)
105. (a) (b) (d)

SECTION 6
Colour Illustrations

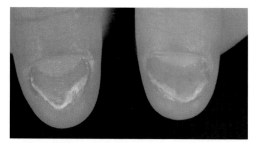

Colour Plate 1. Onycholysis: fingernails showing onycholysis, i.e. separation of the nail from the nail bed. Psoriasis was the explanation in this case; other causes include drugs, fungal infection, trauma and thyrotoxicosis.

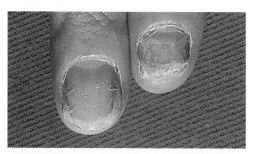

Colour Plate 2. Onychomycosis: fungal infection of the fingernail is not as common as of the toenail, but is suggested here by the thickened crumbling yellowish discoloration of the nail.

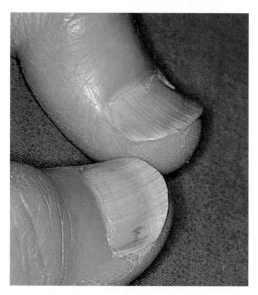

Colour Plate 3. Koilonychia: the characteristic spooning of the fingernails that is a feature of iron-deficiency anaemia is, in fact, rarely seen in clinical practice. (courtesy of Dr. Andrew G. Messenger)

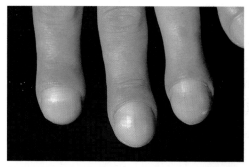

Colour Plate 4. Clubbing: may be congenital or acquired, for example due to respiratory disease, such as bronchial carcinoma or bronchiectasis, or cardiac disorder, such as congenital cyanotic heart defect or infective endocarditis. No underlying problem was found in this case.

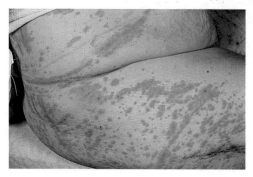

Colour Plate 5. Purpura: bleeding into the skin can produce smaller purpuric lesions (petechiae) or larger areas (ecchymoses). Investigation is needed for a blood disorder, e.g. a low platelet count, absence of a clotting factor or over-treatment with warfarin. (reproduced with permission of Churchill Livingstone)

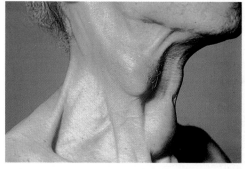

Colour Plate 6. Cervical lymphadenopathy: a search must be made for an underlying malignancy. In this patient, a carcinoma of the piriform fossa was found. A lipoma on the anterior neck is an incidental finding. (courtesy of Mr. Peter D. Bull)

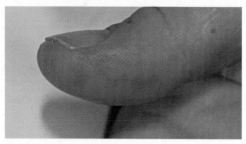

Colour Plate 7. Infective endocarditis: a Janeway lesion is a flat serpiginous lesion on the thenar or hypothenar eminence due to embolism from an infective vegetation. An Osler's node is a firm painful nodule centred on the digit pulp. (courtesy of Dr. Kevin Channer)

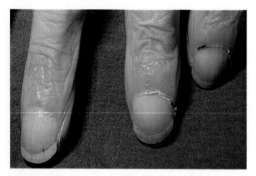

Colour Plate 8. Nailfold infarct with splinter haemorrhage: these changes, which may be seen in infective endocarditis, are due to vasculitis affecting small blood vessels. In this patient, the cause was a vasculitis associated with rheumatoid arthritis. (courtesy of Dr. Mohammed Akil)

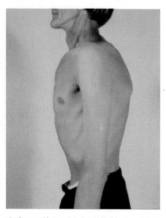

Colour Plate 9. Emphysema of the lungs: the patient is barrel-chested due to hyperinflation of the lungs. (courtesy of Dr. Steve Brennan)

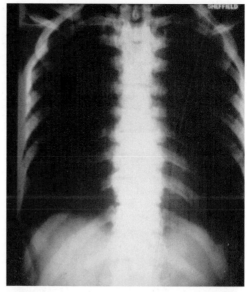

Colour Plate 10. Emphysema of the lung: chest X-ray showing overinflated lungs with a low flat diaphragm. (courtesy of Dr. Steve Brennan)

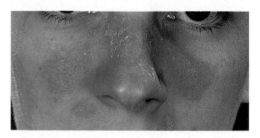

Colour Plate 11. Lupus erythematosus: LE is a multisystem connective tissue disease characterised in many cases by a skin eruption that often affects the face (the so-called 'butterfly rash', which is a photosensitivity eruption).

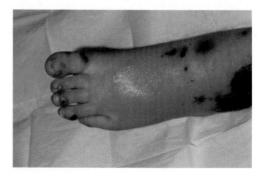

Colour Plate 12. Vasculitis: In vasculitis, circulating immune complexes lodge in the walls of small or medium-sized blood vessels, producing small purpuric lesions that may progress to skin infarcts. Possible causes include drugs, connective tissue diseases, infections and blood disorders.

Gastrointestinal disease

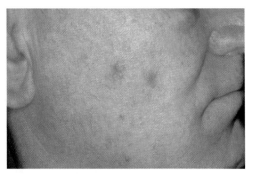

Colour Plate 13. Spider naevi: may be a sign of chronic liver disease, e.g. cirrhosis, which may be the result of excessive alcohol intake. (reproduced with permission of Churchill Livingstone)

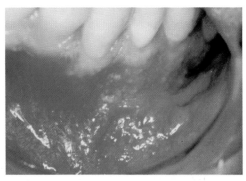

Colour Plate 16. Ulcerative colitis: the condition of pyostomatitis vegetans, characterised by fissuring, pustules and papillary projections, is a rare sign of ulcerative colitis.

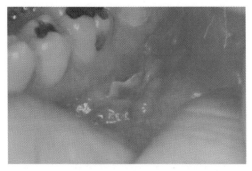

Colour Plate 14. Crohn's disease: thickening and folding of the buccal mucosa, sometimes producing a cobblestone appearance, and associated with granulomatous masses and ulceration, are occasionally seen in Crohn's disease.

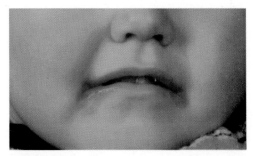

Colour Plate 17. Iron deficiency: an angular stomatitis may be a manifestation of iron deficiency.

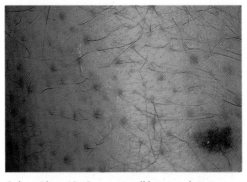

Colour Plate 18. Scurvy: small haemorrhages around hair follicles are illustrated here; other signs found in this patient included bleeding gums, painful joints and woody oedema of the legs.

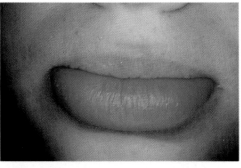

Colour Plate 15. Crohn's disease: granulomatous cheilitis, proven on biopsy of the lip, may be a feature of Crohn's disease.

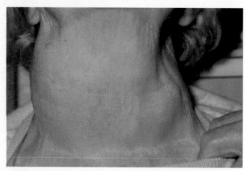

Colour Plate 19. Multinodular goitre: a goitre is visible in this lady. A scar from previous thyroid surgery is evident. She was euthyroid. (courtesy of Dr. Graham Knight)

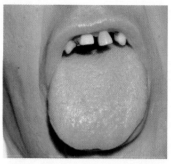

Colour Plate 22. Acromegaly: the characteristic oral changes of macroglossia and widening of the spaces between the teeth are evident in this patient with acromegaly. (courtesy of Dr. Graham Knight)

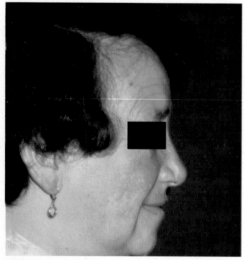

Colour Plate 20. Hypothyroidism: the typical features of puffy skin and hair loss are evident. (courtesy of Dr. Anthony Toft)

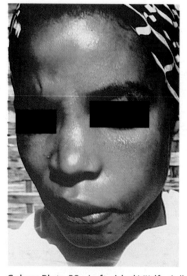

Colour Plate 23. Left-sided VII (facial) nerve palsy: the facial nerve palsy in this patient was due to leprosy. (courtesy of Professor Ross St. C. Barnetson and Gower Medical Publishing)

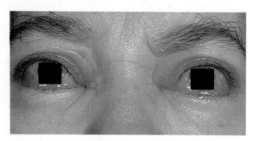

Colour Plate 21. Thyrotoxicosis: this lady, who has an overactive thyroid, has exophthalmos with conjunctivitis. (courtesy of Dr. Graham Knight)

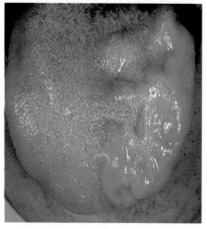

Colour Plate 24. Unilateral XII (hypoglossal) nerve palsy: there is wasting of the left side of the tongue. (reproduced with permission of Gower Medical Publishing)

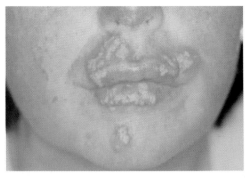

Colour Plate 25. Impetigo: golden crusts, often seen on the face, are characteristic of this condition, which is a superficial infection most often due to *Staphylococcus aureus*.

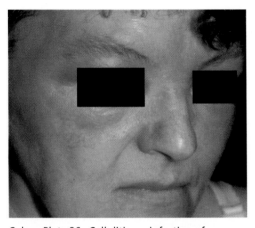

Colour Plate 26. Cellulitis: an infection of the skin and subcutaneous fat, often due to a streptococcal infection, produces a painful swollen appearance associated with a temperature and sometimes rigors. Hospital admission and systemic administration of antibiotics are required.

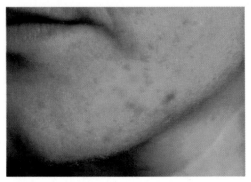

Colour Plate 27. Viral warts: small skin-coloured papules represent plane warts. They often occur on the face.

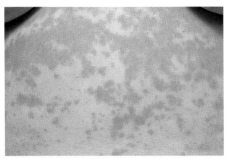

Colour Plate 28. Viral exanthem: the eruption is a blotchy palpable erythema and although non-specific is a frequent accompaniment of a viral infection, especially in children.

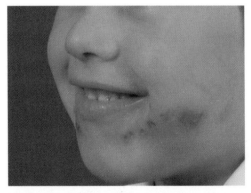

Colour Plate 29. Herpes simplex: 'cold sores' are commonly found on the face, especially around the mouth. They start as blisters that soon break down. Secondary bacterial infection may supervene.

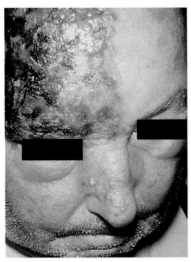

Colour Plate 30. Herpes zoster: 'shingles' is frequently seen in elderly patients and often affects the distribution of the trigeminal nerve, here involving the ophthalmic branch. (reproduced with permission of Churchill Livingstone)

Infectious and allergic disease

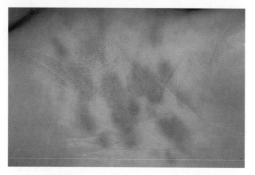

Colour Plate 31. Kaposi's sarcoma: the purplish-brown palpable areas affect the skin or oral mucosa of patients with HIV infection. They are thought to be due to infection with human herpes virus 8. (courtesy of Dr. Andrew G. Messenger)

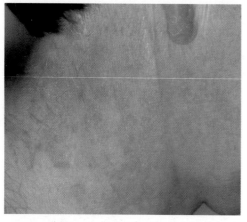

Colour Plate 32. Fungal infection: 'ringworm' classically presents as an expanding annular eruption with central clearing and a scaly raised edge, as illustrated here on the neck.

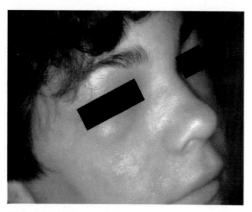

Colour Plate 33. Angioedema: the patient has swelling of the eyelids and face. It may occur due to a food allergy (e.g. to shellfish) but in many cases no underlying cause is found.

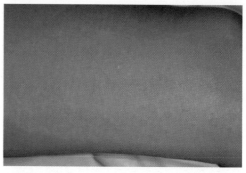

Colour Plate 34. Urticaria: the characteristic red wheals are evident. This pruritic eruption may be due to a food or drug allergy but in most cases of chronic urticaria, no underlying problem is detected.

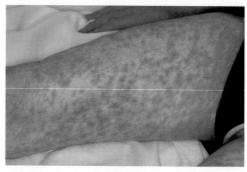

Colour Plate 35. Drug eruption: a rash caused by an allergy to a drug may take a wide variety of forms but typically is maculopapular, as seen in this case on the legs (due to a non-steroidal anti-inflammatory drug).

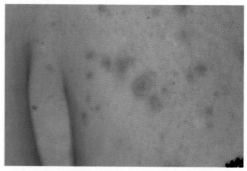

Colour Plate 36. Erythema multiforme: the typical 'target' lesion has a circular red palpable area with a central small blister. Drug hypersensitivity is one cause; others include herpes simplex, streptococcal infection, lupus erythematosus or pregnancy, but quite often, no cause is found.

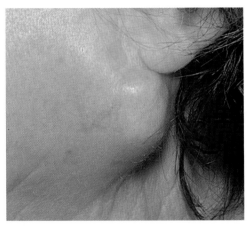

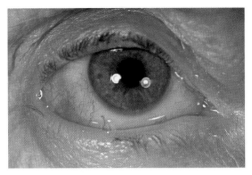

Colour Plate 40. Mucous membrane pemphigoid: mucous membrane pemphigoid is a scarring bullous disorder that can affect the ocular and oral mucosa. Scarring and the formation of conjunctival adhesions can be seen.

Colour Plate 37. Parotid tumour: this tumour usually presents as a slow-growing well-defined firm mass in the parotid gland at the angle of the jaw. Assessment and removal by an ENT surgeon is required. (courtesy of Mr. Peter D. Bull)

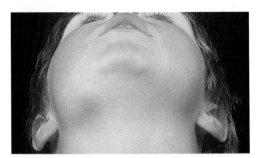

Colour Plate 38. Swollen submandibular gland: a swelling in the right submandibular salivary gland in this child is due to infection with an atypical mycobacterium. (courtesy of Mr. Peter D. Bull)

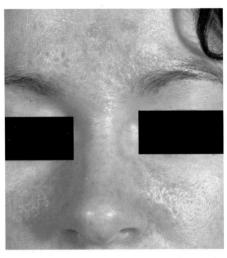

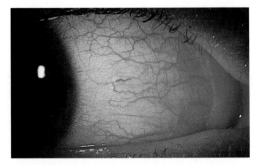

Colour Plate 41. Facial eczema: a scaly eruption of the face can be due to an endogenous dermatitis, e.g. atopic eczema, or – as in this case – seborrhoeic dermatitis in which the central part of the face is involved, or an exogenous contact dermatitis.

Colour Plate 39. Red eye: the problem of 'red eye' may be due to a variety of ophthalmic disorders. In this case, the patient has acute iritis. (courtesy of Mr. Som Prasad)

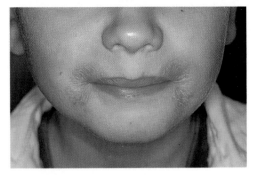

Colour Plate 42. Contact dermatitis: an inflammatory eruption due to allergy or irritancy to an external substance in contact with the skin is characteristic of contact dermatitis. In this child, this was due to a fragrance in an over-the-counter moisturising cream.

Skin disease

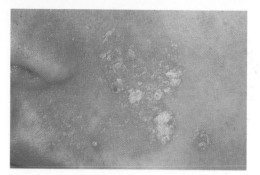

Colour Plate 43. Psoriasis: it is not common for psoriasis to affect the face but when it occurs, as in this man, it is characterised by redness and scaling.

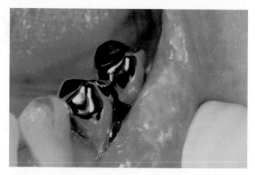

Colour Plate 46. Oral lichen planus: in some cases oral lichen planus is due to contact allergy to mercury from amalgam restorations or, less commonly, from gold in a capped tooth, as shown in this patient.

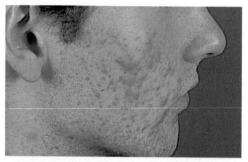

Colour Plate 44. Acne: acne is a frequent eruption in adolescents, and is characterised by blackheads, pustules and cysts on the face (and also on the back and chest).

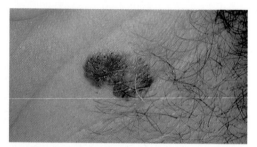

Colour Plate 47. Malignant melanoma: malignant melanoma is a serious skin cancer with metastatic potential. In this patient, the tumour shows variability in pigmentation and outline: it was excised with appropriate margins and the diagnosis confirmed. (reproduced with permission of Churchill Livingstone)

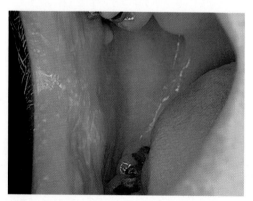

Colour Plate 45. Oral lichen planus: white lace-like areas on the buccal mucosa typically characterise oral lichen planus. There may be cutaneous lesions elsewhere.

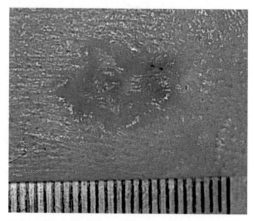

Colour Plate 48. Basal cell carcinoma: basal cell carcinomas are commonly found on the face. There are different types. The one shown here on the forehead is of the scarring (morphoeic) type.

Index